A Reference Manual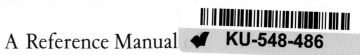

Growth and Development

A Reference Manual of Growth and Development

J. M. H. BUCKLER

MA, DM, FRCP
Senior Lecturer, Department of
Paediatrics and Child Health,
University of Leeds;
Honorary Consultant Paediatrician,
Leeds Area Health Authority (Teaching)

BLACKWELL
SCIENTIFIC PUBLICATIONS
OXFORD LONDON EDINBURGH
MELBOURNE

© 1979 Blackwell Scientific Publications
Osney Mead, Oxford OX2 0EL
8 John Street, London WC1N 2ES
9 Forrest Road, Edinburgh EH1 2QH
P.O. Box 9, North Balwyn, Victoria, Australia

First published 1979

Buckler, J M H
    A reference manual of growth and development.
    1. Children — Growth — Statistics
    I. Title
    612.6'5'0212   RJ131
    ISBN 0–632–00185–2

Distributed in the USA by
Blackwell Mosby Book Distributors
11830 Westline Industrial Drive
St. Louis, Missouri 63141
and in Canada by
Blackwell Mosby Book Distributors
86 Northline Road, Toronto
Ontario, M4B 3E5

Set by Hope Services, Clifton Hampden and
printed in Great Britain by
Express Litho Service (Oxford)
and bound by
Kemp Hall Bindery, Oxford

Contents

Acknowledgements

In compiling this book, I acknowledge with gratitude the many individuals named in the relevant places in the text who have allowed me to reproduce their data. In particular, I express appreciation to Professor J.M. Tanner whose material constitutes the basis for a large proportion of this manual, and from whom I have received much help and advice over the years. I am particularly grateful to Professor R.W. Smithells for his continual support, encouragement and advice in every aspect of the preparation of this book, and to Miss Janet Hall for her invaluable secretarial work. I also thank Professor D.

Jackson, for his help in writing the chapter on dental development, Dr. S.R. Meadow and Miss Valerie Pomfret for comments and advice about developmental assessment, and Dr. Olive Scott for reviewing the chapter on Electrocardiography.

Figures 4.1–4.8, 5.1–5.4, 6.1–6.4, 7.1–7.4, 8.1–8.4 and 12.3–12.4, prepared by Professor J.M. Tanner and Mr. R.H. Whitehouse and Figures 12.1–12.2 prepared by Dr. D. Gairdner and Dr. J. Pearson, are reproduced by permission of Castlemead Publications, Hertford.

Introduction

Normal infants and children never remain static in their physical and mental characteristics due to a continuing process of growth and development. Interpretation of such characteristics in children is of fundamental importance, in contrast to adults in whom changes related to growth are minimal. Before any attempt can be made to recognise or evaluate an abnormal state, it is essential to have a knowledge of the normal physical and developmental changes occurring as a child grows up.

There are many references to normal data available on children, but the purpose of this volume is to present such material from reliable sources in a compact, convenient form handy for quick reference, and restricted to those pieces of information likely to be most frequently required by medical practitioners dealing with children. Data are presented mainly in the form of charts and tables and represent normal values with an indication of the range which may be expected within the population concerned. This population is usually British and data may not be appropriate for other nations or races. The nature of the population from which the data were derived can be found from the references. Brief comments are included as explanation and to aid in application. Little reference is made to causes or diagnosis of abnormal conditions, and the manual does not include normal values for laboratory investigations.

1: Identification of the normal

Centile distributions and normality

The distribution of values for a measurement within a population is conveniently shown on centile charts. A position on a centile chart indicates the proportion of the population whose measurement at the same age is greater or smaller than that of the subject. This, however, only gives limited information regarding the likelihood that this subject's measurements may be considered normal or within the normal range. The concept of 'normality' in itself needs defining as some may interpret this entirely on the basis of population distribution, whereas to most it implies good general health and appropriate development. Though positions near the mean are more likely to be normal and extreme centile positions to be abnormal, many other factors must be taken into account, and conclusions based on these observations alone may well be misleading. Values which correspond most closely to the mean are not necessarily optimal values. This would imply that the population as a whole has optimal proportions and this is not always so, as illustrated by the high proportion of overweight individuals within Western populations which has resulted in a skew of the centile distribution for weight. Many measurements such as height or intelligence quotient conform to a Gaussian distribution in healthy populations and for these centile positions can be related to standard deviations (S.D.) as indicated in Figure 1.1. In such cases, the 97th and 3rd centile lines approximately correspond to ± 2 S.D. from the mean. Standard deviations require a Gaussian distribution for application whereas centile distributions do not, and measurements such as weight or skinfold thicknesses which do not have a normal distribution cannot be conveniently referred to in terms of standard deviations.

Accuracy of measurements

Inaccurate measurements may be misleading. A small error in a single observation which is unlikely to be repeated subsequently may give adequate information, but in assessing ongoing progress inaccuracies render the serial measurements of little value. Ideally sequential measurements should be taken by the same observer under the same circumstances including the time of day and the use of the same technique. Unfortunately this is not always practicable, but recog-

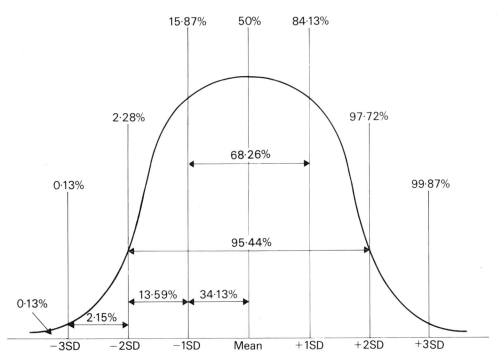

Figure 1.1. Relationship between centiles and standard deviations for values with a Gaussian distribution.

nition of the limitations which such deficiencies impose, and restricting them to a minimum by using correct techniques, will make interpretation more meaningful. Changes in many measurements, such as length and height, are slow, so that there is little value in repeating them at short time intervals, as the true change may not be far different from the error of measurement. Other values such as weight may change significantly much more rapidly, and will need interpreting in a different light.

Basic criteria of normality and indices of abnormality

Certain guidelines in interpretation of centile positions are helpful.

(a) Position on the centile chart

Clearly, as indicated above, the nearer to the mean position the more likely is a measurement to be normal, and the further away the more likely to be abnormal. Frequently this alone forms the basis on which fuller evaluation is undertaken. Values above 97th or below 3rd centiles frequently are accepted as indications for further assessment.

(b) Relationship between centile positions of different physical parameters

In general the centile positions of various body measurements, such as height and weight, will be approximately the same in a normal child, and a gross difference in one from another may well be significant.

(c) Deviation of serial measurements from centile lines

Longitudinal data, if accurate, are much more informative than single measurements. Serial measurements which deviate from a centile line are more commonly associated with pathology than those which adhere to a constant centile line. This applies particularly to measurements based primarily on bone structure where a long term disorder is required to produce a significant effect. Others, such as weight or skinfold thickness may fluctuate much more rapidly, sometimes with negative velocities, without necessarily indicating disease. Deviations from centile lines around the age of puberty must clearly be evaluated with reference to the stage of pubertal development.

(d) Similarity of family pattern

Among the normal influences on growth are familial factors, the significance of which should never be ignored. A knowledge of the body proportions and features of parents and siblings throws much light on the significance of such observations in the child concerned. Measurements outside the normal centile distribution may well be explained in terms of the family pattern, although the occasional occurrence of an inherited or common environmental pathology should not be forgotten. Whether or not a child's height can be accounted for by the heights of the parents depends on the relative centile positions of these measurements. Charts have been prepared in which children's heights can be evaluated in terms of parental heights (Tanner et al. 1970; see Appendix), but in practice it is as easy and almost as reliable to compare the child's centile position with the mean of those of the parents as estimated from the adult standards on the height centile charts for the appropriate sexes.

(e) Population variations

Centile charts are only appropriate for the population from which they were derived. Many of the charts shown here are based on various studies by Tanner et al. of children in Oxford, London and Harpenden mainly before 1960. Their values may not apply to populations from different regions, countries or races, and there is an additional error due to secular change. These factors should be taken into consideration in interpreting centile positions, though gross aberrations from normal positions are hardly likely to be misinterpreted.

2: Units of measurement

Linear and weight measurements

In these tables and charts, measurements are usually given in both metric and non-metric values. Despite the advantages of the metric system, many physicians and most lay people will continue for some time to be more familiar with feet, inches, pounds and ounces, and it will be necessary to convert to and from these values.

A conversion table for heights and weights is included in the surface area nomogram in Figure 2.2.

Ages

These will be recorded both in terms of years and months and in decimals of years. Figure 2.1 shows the days of the year in terms of decimal dates. For doctors in most circumstances it is easier and more practical to consider ages in terms of years and months. However, in evaluating changes in measurements and velocities of growth, the decimal system is essential. In computing decimal dates, the year is divided into tenths, not twelfths (months), and each day of the year is ascribed a value, as indicated in the figure 2.1, in terms of thousandths of the year. The decimal age is calculated by direct subtraction of the decimal birth date from the decimal date of examination. The time interval between examinations is the direct subtraction between two decimal dates or ages.

	1 JAN.	2 FEB.	3 MAR.	4 APR.	5 MAY	6 JUNE	7 JULY	8 AUG.	9 SEPT.	10 OCT.	11 NOV.	12 DEC.
1	000	085	162	247	329	414	496	581	666	748	833	915
2	003	088	164	249	332	416	499	584	668	751	836	918
3	005	090	167	252	334	419	501	586	671	753	838	921
4	008	093	170	255	337	422	504	589	674	756	841	923
5	011	096	173	258	340	425	507	592	677	759	844	926
6	014	099	175	260	342	427	510	595	679	762	847	929
7	016	101	178	263	345	430	512	597	682	764	849	932
8	019	104	181	266	348	433	515	600	685	767	852	934
9	022	107	184	268	351	436	518	603	688	770	855	937
10	025	110	186	271	353	438	521	605	690	773	858	940
11	027	112	189	274	356	441	523	608	693	775	860	942
12	030	115	192	277	359	444	526	611	696	778	863	945
13	033	118	195	279	362	447	529	614	699	781	866	948
14	036	121	197	282	364	449	532	616	701	784	868	951
15	038	123	200	285	367	452	534	619	704	786	871	953
16	041	126	203	288	370	455	537	622	707	789	874	956
17	044	129	205	290	373	458	540	625	710	792	877	959
18	047	132	208	293	375	460	542	627	712	795	879	962
19	049	134	211	296	378	463	545	630	715	797	882	964
20	052	137	214	299	381	466	548	633	718	800	885	967
21	055	140	216	301	384	468	551	636	721	803	888	970
22	058	142	219	304	386	471	553	638	723	805	890	973
23	060	145	222	307	389	474	556	641	726	808	893	975
24	063	148	225	310	392	477	559	644	729	811	896	978
25	066	151	227	312	395	479	562	647	731	814	899	981
26	068	153	230	315	397	482	564	649	734	816	901	984
27	071	156	233	318	400	485	567	652	737	819	904	986
28	074	159	236	321	403	488	570	655	740	822	907	989
29	077		238	323	405	490	573	658	742	825	910	992
30	079		241	326	408	493	575	660	745	827	912	995
31	082		244		411		578	663		830		997
	JAN. 1	FEB. 2	MAR. 3	APR. 4	MAY 5	JUNE 6	JULY 7	AUG. 8	SEPT. 9	OCT. 10	NOV. 11	DEC. 12

Figure 2.1 Table of decimals of year.

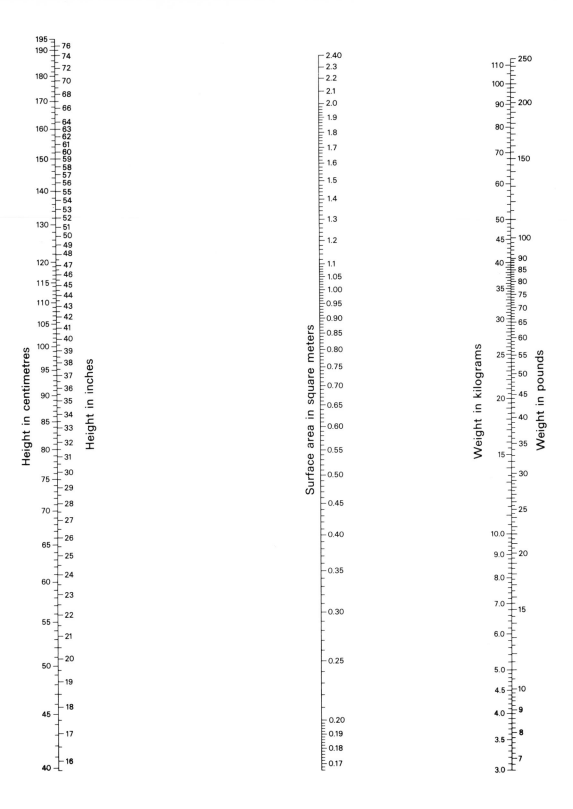

Figure 2.2 Surface area nomogram. (Extracted from *Documenta Geigy Scientific Tables*, 7th edition, Basle, 1970. Courtesy Ciba-Geigy Limited, Basle, Switzerland.)

3: Surface area

As a reference standard, surface area is frequently more appropriate than height, weight or age. This may, for example, be the case in determining drug dosage or potential overdosage, and in estimating basal metabolism and metabolic requirements, fluid and electrolyte losses and replacement requirements, particularly in burns. Surface area is easily calculated by means of a nomogram, shown in Figure 2.2 by finding where the line joining the appropriate height and weight values for the child crosses the surface area column.

For older children and adults an approximate method of assessing surface area percentage involvement in a skin lesion, such as a burn, uses the 'Rule of 9s'. The body surface area can be roughly divided into 9 equal units, 1 for head and neck, 1 for each arm, 2 for each leg and 2 for the trunk. However, this method cannot be applied in young children, whose body proportions are different from those of adults. An approximate indication of surface area proportions of body components at different ages is shown in Figure 3.1. This indicates that though the head and legs alter greatly in the proportions of the body which they contribute, the trunk and arms remain relatively constant throughout the growing years.

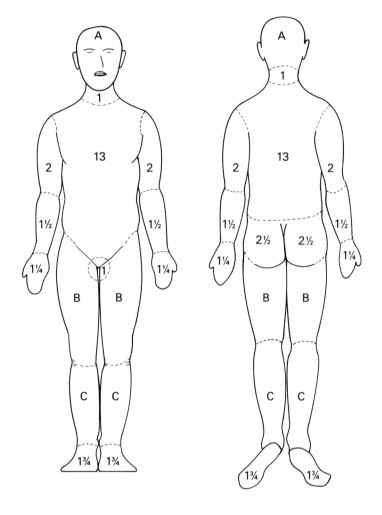

Age	A = ½ of head	B = ½ of one thigh	C = ½ of lower leg
0	9½	2¾	2½
1	8½	3¼	2½
5	6½	4	2¾
10	5½	4¼	3
15	4½	4½	3¼
Adult	3½	4¾	3½

Figure 3.1 Relative percentages of surface area according to age.

4: Length, height and weight

Technique of measurement

These are based on the descriptions of Tanner *et al.* (1969).

Standing height and supine length

Serial measurements should ideally be undertaken by the same observer. In practice this is often not possible, but those undertaking measurements should be trained staff familiar with a standard technique. Measurements of height and length should be recorded to the nearest 0.1 cm. Measurement of length is greater than that of stature by up to 1 cm in any one subject, and it should be recorded which of these measurements was taken. The customary age for changing the method of measurement from length to height is between 2 and 3 years, depending on the child's ability to cooperate.

Height

This is preferably measured with a stadiometer (Harpenden) but often a rule fixed vertically to a wall, and with a smoothly sliding horizontal head-piece, is used as a cheaper alternative. An anthropometer may be used for measuring height in field studies. The subject, without shoes, stands as tall and straight as possible, ensuring that the heels maintain contact with the ground, and the back and heels are in contact with the wall or stadiometer. Head tilt is avoided by instructing the child to look straight ahead, which should bring the lower margin of the eye socket to the same level as the external auditory meatus. The child is then stretched gently by upward pressure under the mastoid processes and instructed to relax the shoulders so that these are not shrugged. The sliding headpiece is lowered to rest firmly on the head and the measurement read directly off the sliding scale or the rule on the wall to the nearest millimetre.

Length

This is measured using a firm horizontal board with a fixed vertical head-piece and a smooth sliding vertical foot-piece (e.g. Harpenden neonatometer or Harpenden infant measuring table). The scale is either along the length of the board or a sliding scale on the foot-piece. The infant is laid supine and one observer holds the head against the head board, maintaining the head in line with the body. The other observer stretches the legs, ensuring that they and the body are straight and, holding the feet at right angles to the legs, brings the sliding footpiece into gentle but firm contact with the heels and soles. Length is recorded to the nearest millimetre.

Weight

Babies and children should be weighed in the nude or with light underclothes. Serial measurements should preferably be made on the same scales. Babies are laid on a dry cloth (for which weight correction is made) in the pan of a balance. Older children stand on balance scales, but must not touch the upright of the scale or any other objects alongside. Sometimes with difficult younger children it is easier for weight to be ascertained as the difference between the weights of an adult holding the child and then standing alone. Weights can be recorded to the nearest 0.1 kg, greater accuracy than this being without value in view of the marked weight changes in normal children from day to day under the same circumstances (Rao and Sastry 1976).

Length or height centiles, with the corresponding weight centiles for the various age groups 0–5 years and 0–19 years, are shown for boys in Figures 4.1* to 4.4 and for girls in Figures 4.5 to 4.8, based on the data of Tanner *et al.* (1966), Tanner and Whitehouse (1973 and 1976). Reference may also be made to Figures 12.1 and 12.2, which combine, for boys and girls respectively, length, weight and height circumference centiles up to the age of 2 years, including a correction for the duration of gestation (Gairdner and Pearson 1971). A similar correction is also included in Figures 4.1 and 4.2, and in 4.5 and 4.6.

*The figures in this chapter are based on the standards presented by Tanner J.M., Whitehouse R.H. and Takaishi M. (1966) *Archives of Disease in Childhood*, **41**, 454 and 613 and are reproduced by permission of the authors and editors. Tanner J.M. and Whitehouse R.H. (1973) *Archives of Disease in Childhood*, **48**, 786, Tanner J.M. and Whitehouse R.H. (1976) *Archives of Disease in Childhood*, **51**, 170.

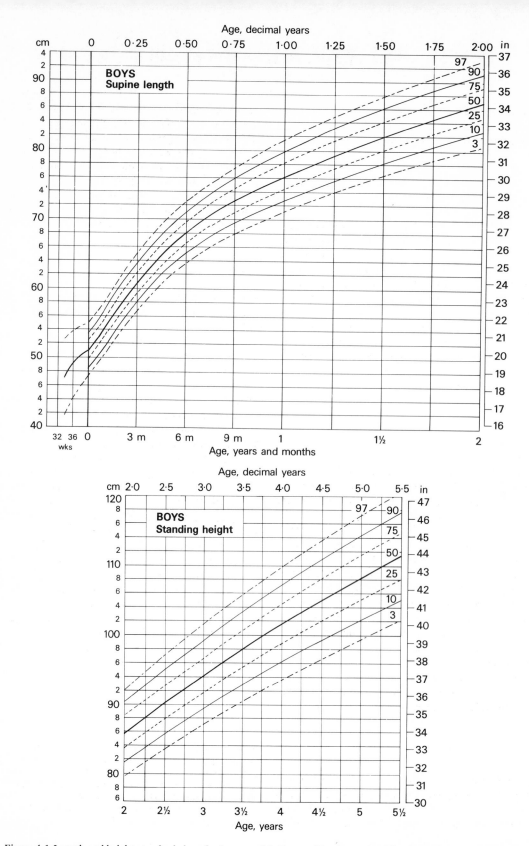

Figure 4.1 Length and height standard chart for boys aged 0–5 years (Castlemead Publications Chart No. SHWB 28).

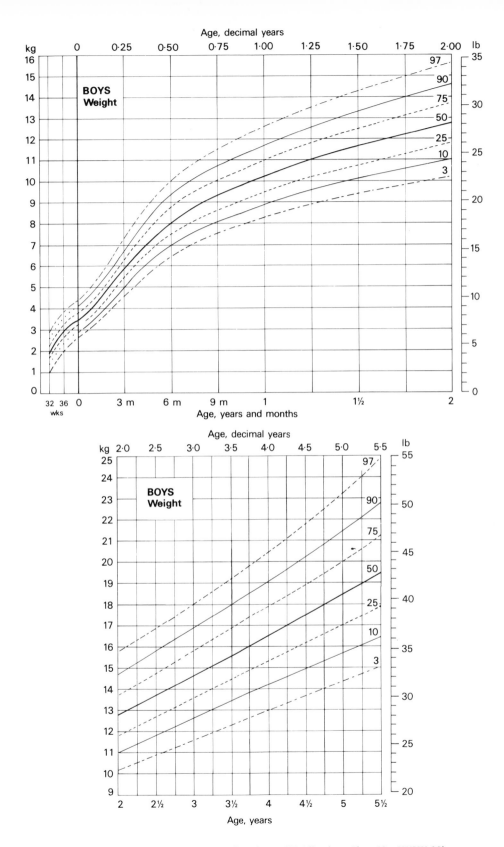

Figure 4.2 Weight standard chart for boys aged 0–5 years (Castlemead Publications Chart No. XXXX 00).

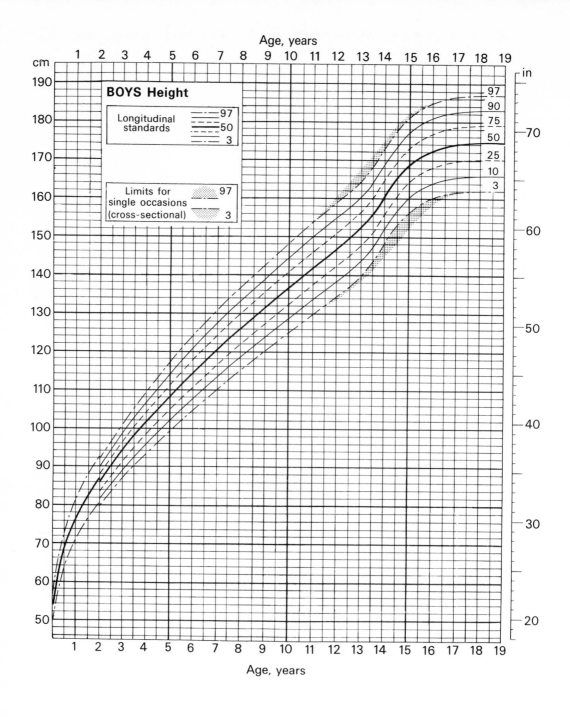

Figure 4.3 Height standard chart for boys aged 0–19 years (Castlemead Publications Chart No. GDB11A).

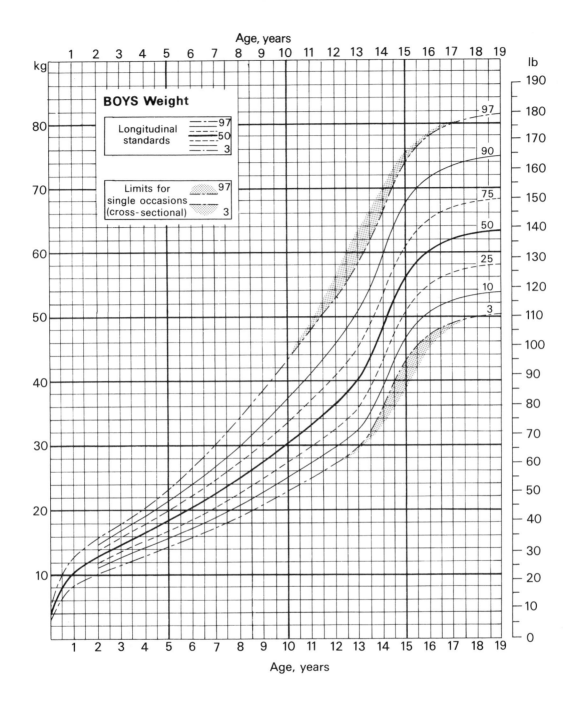

Figure 4.4 Weight standard chart for boys aged 0–19 years (Castlemead Publications Chart No. GDB11A).

13

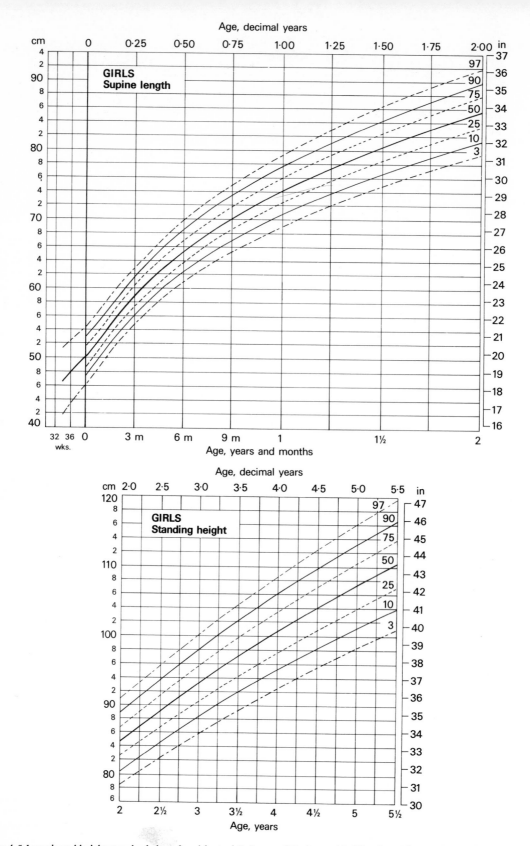

Figure 4.5 Length and height standard chart for girls aged 0–5 years (Castlemead Publications Chart No. SHWG29).

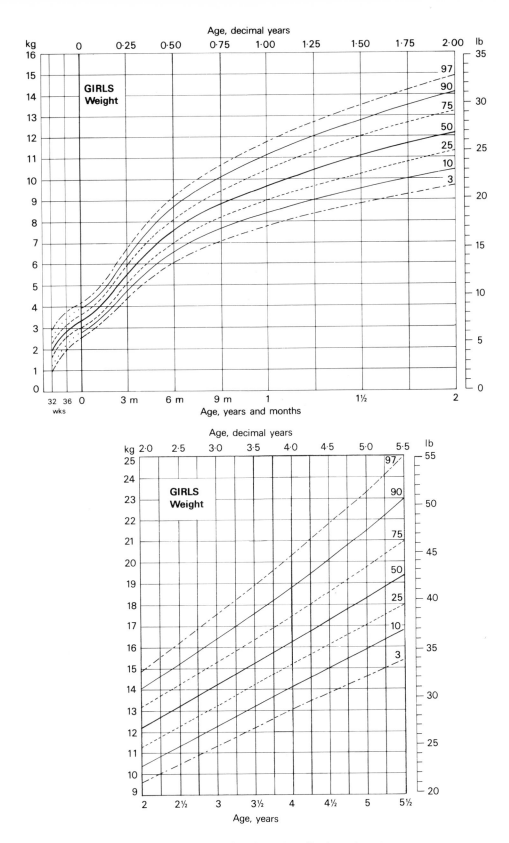

Figure 4.6 Weight standard chart for girls aged 0–5 years (Castlemead Publications Chart No. SHWG29).

15

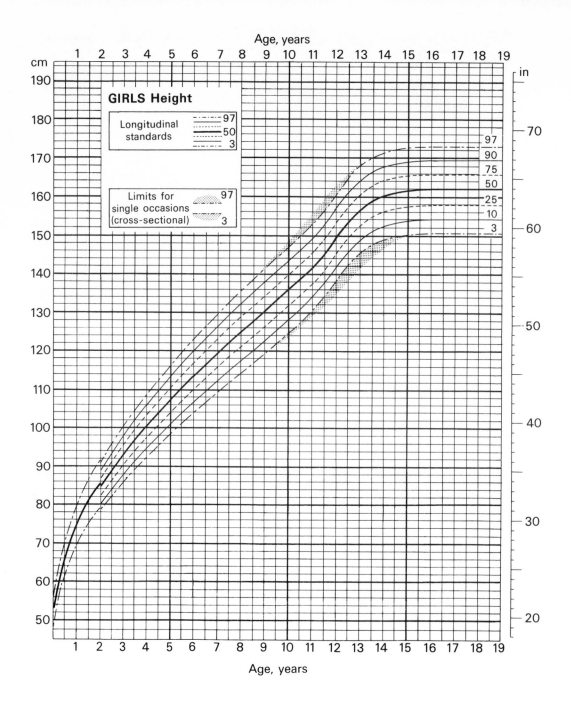

Figure 4.7 Height standard chart for girls aged 0–19 years (Castlemead Publications Chart No. GDG12A).

16

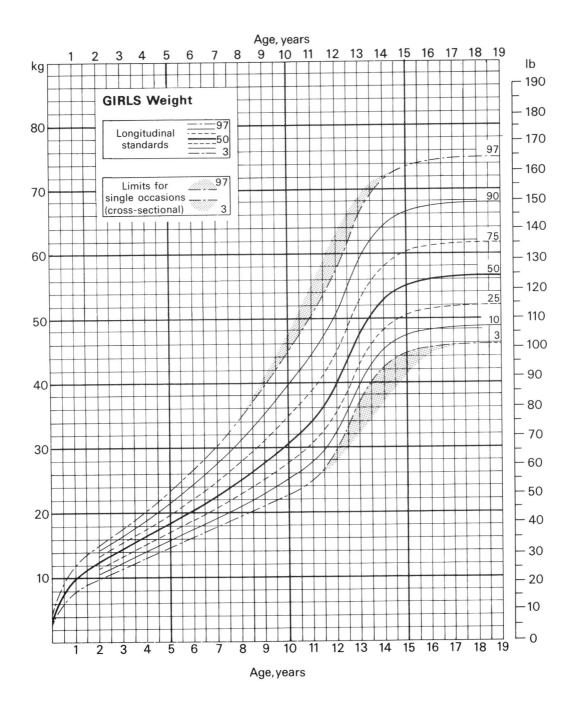

Figure 4.8 Weight standard chart for girls aged 0–19 years (Castlemead Publications Chart No. GDG12A).

5: Height and weight velocity

Method of estimation

Growth velocities are recorded as changes in measurements over a period of a year. Estimation of velocities is easier if time intervals are considered as decimals of a year. Height velocities are always positive values, but as weight may be lost, weight velocities could be negative. Whereas linear centiles reflect predominantly what has happened in the past, velocities show changes relating only to the time around that of the recording. Velocities may be estimated in two different ways.

(a) Differences in whole year measurements

The difference in height or weight over a period of a year is recorded as the velocity at the midpoint between these times. (It is unlikely that the interval will be exactly a year, but a simple correction may be applied for the precise age difference). The subject will probably be measured at more frequent intervals, but after a year the annual differences can be repeatedly used in this way for plotting on the velocity chart, so giving more frequent velocity records than once every year.

(b) Differences in measurements over shorter time intervals

The rate of growth in terms of a full year period is estimated by multiplying the short term growth over a known interval by the appropriate time factor, as if that growth rate had continued for a full year. Consecutive growth rates in terms of the growth per year can be recorded at the mid-point in time between each of these measurements.

Interpretation

Before puberty, the average growth velocity centile position over a long period for any one healthy child adheres much more closely to the mean than may occur with linear centiles. A normal child's growth pattern will frequently follow a particular linear centile line over the years, be it the 3rd or 97th, but to do this requires an overall velocity that lies much closer to the 50th velocity centile line and consistent adherence to 3rd or 97th velocity lines will result in progressive deviation from a linear centile. This does not apply at periods of rapid growth, notably at puberty, for the great variation in the age at which this normally occurs will cause this line to be shifted earlier or later than the mean age position illustrated on the charts. Though the shape of the height velocity curve may vary in the magnitude of the peak and the broadness of its duration, these variations are not as marked as the variations in the ages at which the accelerated growth may occur. Nevertheless, early maturers tend to have greater peak height velocities and late maturers peak values which are less than those of children who mature at an average age. These differences are much less striking in girls than in boys and are also less marked in velocity curves for weight than for height.

Over short periods variations in velocities may be considerable in normal healthy children, e.g. seasonal variations (Marshall 1971), and interpreting these data in terms of growth over a year may be misleading. Intervals between measurements must be sufficiently long for growth to be significant and well in excess of the possible error of the measurement, which will be multiplied when velocities in yearly terms are based on these values. There is little merit in working out height velocities over periods of less than 3 months (except at puberty), and for weight short-term changes may be very different from the long-term overall pattern.

However, relatively short duration changes related to disease processes and the ensuing catch up of growth may not be apparent when evaluated in terms of measurement differences at yearly intervals. Also, the precise pattern of growth through puberty will appear very differently depending on the method of assessment, as velocity changes will alter from month to month and the peak growth rate may only extend over a few months. Growth evaluated in terms of annual differences will flatten this curve considerably.

However, apart from the dramatic rapid changes at puberty and relatively short-lasting disease processes, longitudinal growth studies will produce a more meaningful velocity pattern if based on annual differences. The precise method of assessing velocities will therefore depend on the particular clinical circumstances.

Value of Velocity Recordings

1   Recognition of a consistent deviation from the mean height and weight velocity range as an indication of possible underlying pathology.

2   Demonstration of response to treatment as catch-up (accelerated) velocity, or occasionally decelerated velocity.

3   In the monitoring of growth at puberty, relating the growth spurt to chronological age and to the other changes of puberty (of particular value in correlating tall and short stature to the pubertal status).

Velocity centile charts for height and weight are shown for boys in Figures 5.1* and 5.2, and for girls in Figures 5.3 and 5.4 (Tanner and Whitehouse 1976). These figures include an indication of the different patterns of velocity curves for early and late developers, showing the range which may be found in those whose peak velocities occur up to 2 standard deviations before or after the mean age.

*All figures in this chapter are based on the standards presented by Tanner J. M., Whitehouse R. H., and Takaishi M. (1966) *Archives of Disease in Childhood*, **41**, 454 and 613, and described further by Tanner J. M. and Whitehouse R. H. (1976) *Archives of Disease in Childhood*, **51**, 170, and reproduced by permission of the authors and editors.

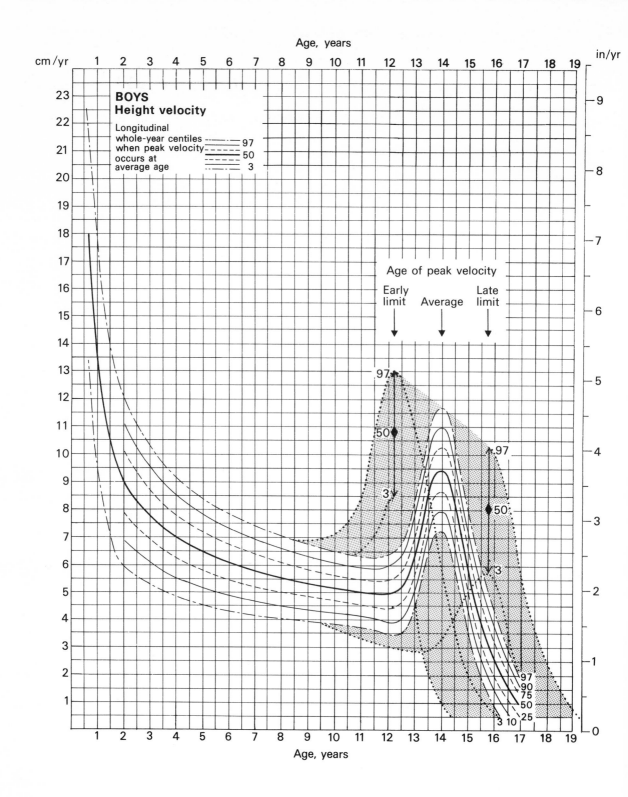

Figure 5.1 Height velocity centile chart for boys (Castlemead Publications Chart No. LBHV2A).

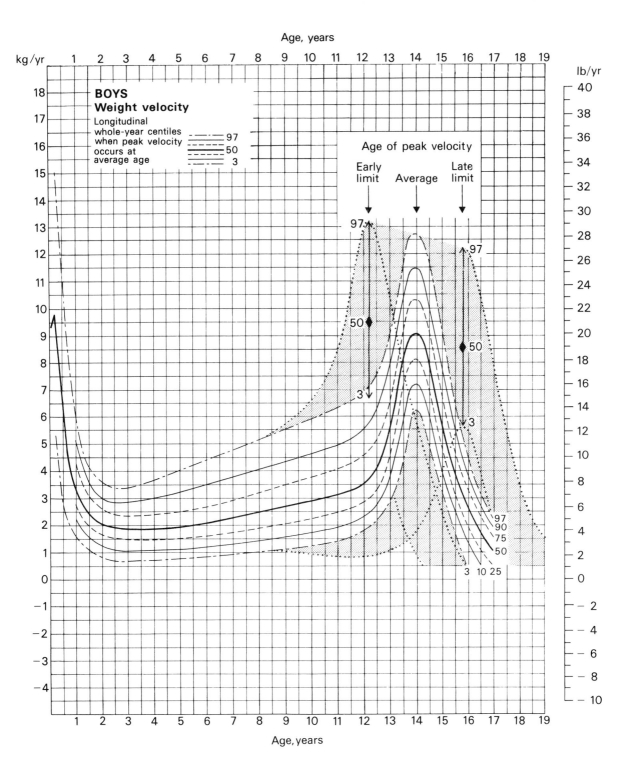

Figure 5.2 Weight velocity centile chart for boys (Castlemead Publications Chart No. LBWV6A).

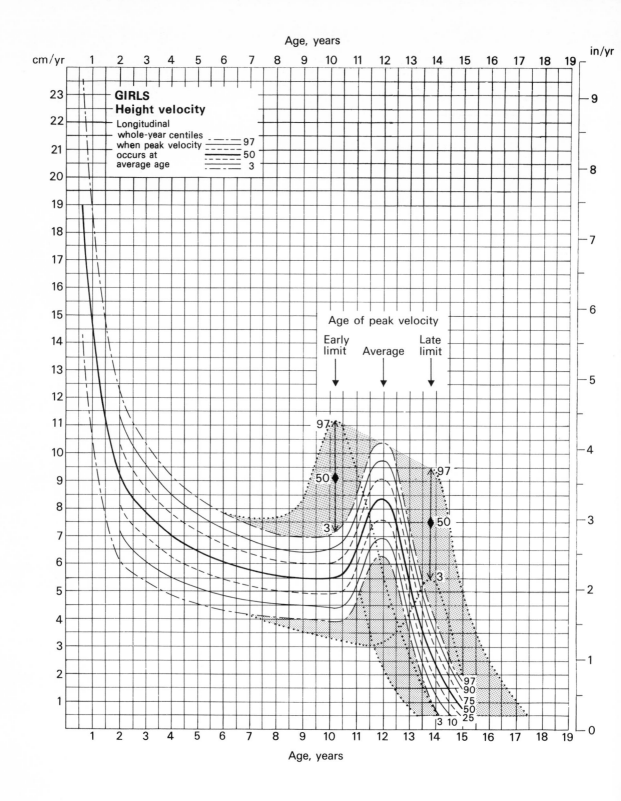

Figure 5.3 Height velocity centile chart for girls (Castlemead Publications Chart No. LGHV4A).

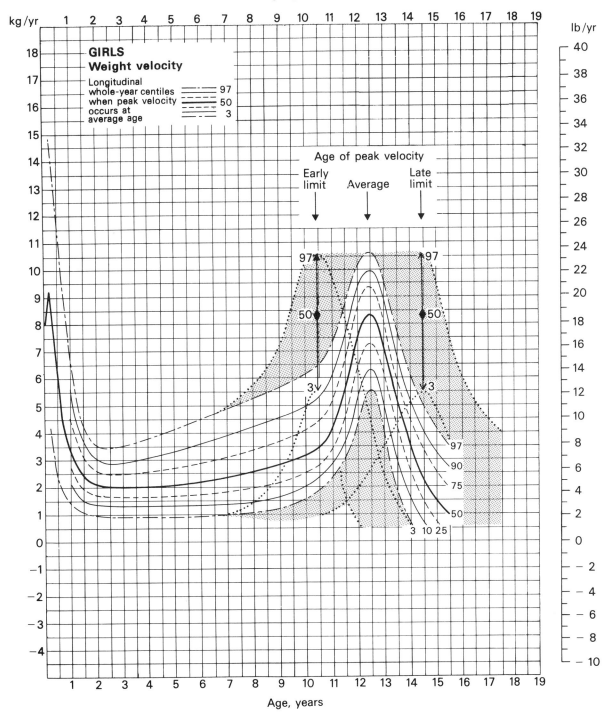

Figure 5.4 Weight velocity centile chart for girls (Castlemead Publications Chart No. LGWV8A).

6: Sitting height

Technique of Measurement

Sitting height is measured with an anthropometer (Harpenden). The child sits on a flat table with the backs of his knees in contact with the edge of the table, over which the legs hang loosely. He sits as tall and straight as possible, but with shoulders relaxed and avoiding tilting of the head. Measurement is made with the anthropometer accurately vertical and in contact with the sacrum, the spine between the shoulders and the back of the head, and gentle traction is applied upwards to the chin. Correct positioning may be more reliably achieved if a second observer stands behind the subject. The horizontal arm of the anthropometer is brought to rest on the top of the head and the sitting height is read directly from the sliding scale.

In young children a comparable measurement, crown-rump, can be obtained using a horizontal length measurement board. The child lies flat on his back, but with his legs held vertically at the hips by one observer. Another observer holds the head under gentle traction in contact with the fixed head piece, while the other brings the movable foot piece with sliding scale in contact with the buttocks.

Interpretation

Centile charts for sitting height (and crown-rump measurements) are shown for boys and girls in Figures 6.1* and 6.3.*

Sitting height measurements provide a useful substitute for height in children who cannot stand, or who have congenital defects of the legs. In other individuals the relationship of sitting height to full stature gives information similar to, though more accurate than, that provided by the ratio of upper to lower segments or comparison of stature to span.

Comparison of the centile positions for sitting height and full stature from the appropriate charts will give an indication of whether or not leg and trunk proportions are normal for age, and so aid in the recognition of various bone dysplasias, anomalies of limbs and in differentiation of endocrine disorders affecting growth. Before puberty and in early puberty growth is predominantly in the limbs, whereas in the later stages of growth trunk lengthening is more evident. When puberty is earlier or later than average, this may be reflected in limb to trunk proportions that are atypical for a chronological age but will be appropriate for the stage of puberty; though in certain extreme or pathological situations of early or delayed puberty an abnormality of limb proportion may persist.

More precise correlations between limb and trunk proportions can be obtained using Figures 6.2† and 6.4† for boys and girls respectively. These plot separately on the same chart sitting height (or crown-rump measurement) and subischial leg length (or rump-heel measurement) which is estimated as stature minus sitting height. The graphs indicate standard deviations for these measurements.

*Based on the data of Tanner J. M. and Whitehouse R. H.
†These figures are based on data to be presented by Tanner J. M. and Whitehouse R. H. in *Atlas of Children's Growth*, to be published by Academic Press, London in 1979, by permission of the authors.

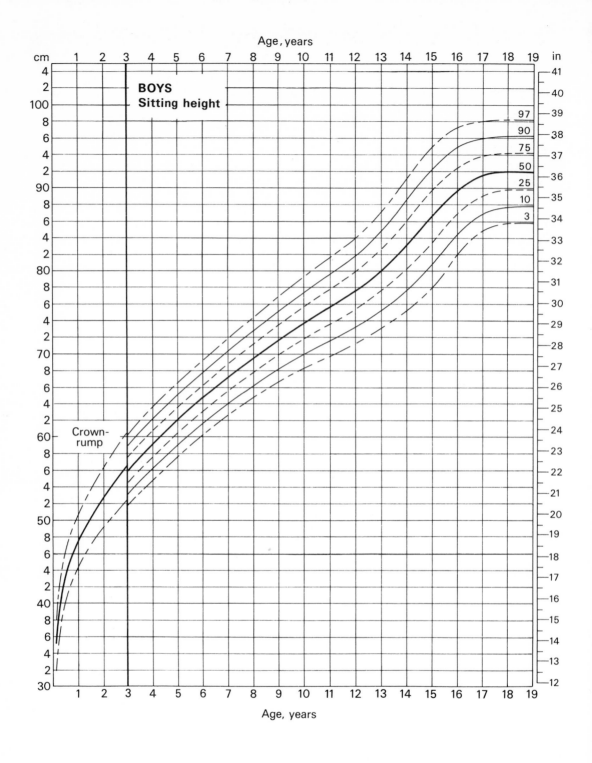

Figure 6.1 Centile chart for sitting height (and crown–rump measurement) for boys (˙stlemead Publications Chart No. SHB21).

26

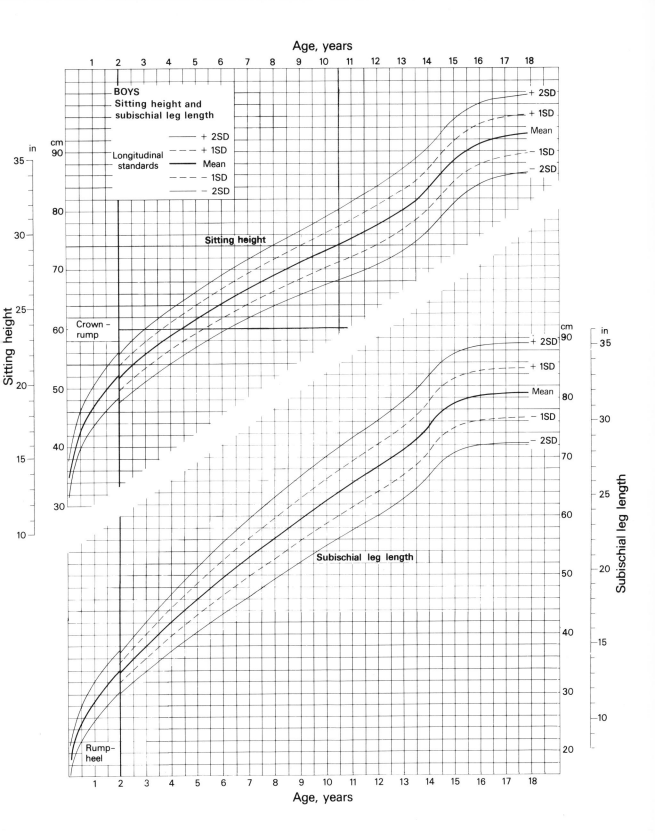

Figure 6.2 Centile chart relating sitting height and subischial leg length in boys (Castlemead Publications Chart No. LSHB51).

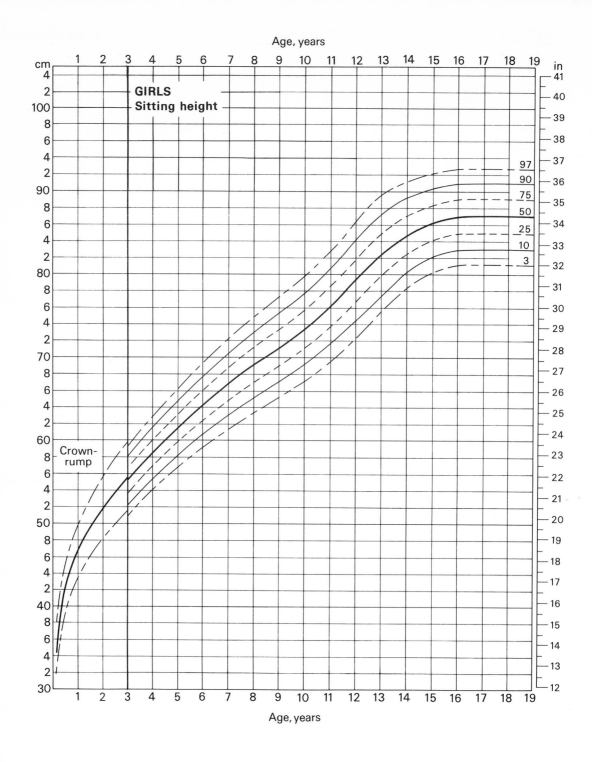

Figure 6.3 Centile chart for sitting height (and crown–rump measurement) for girls (Castlemead Publications Chart No. SHG22).

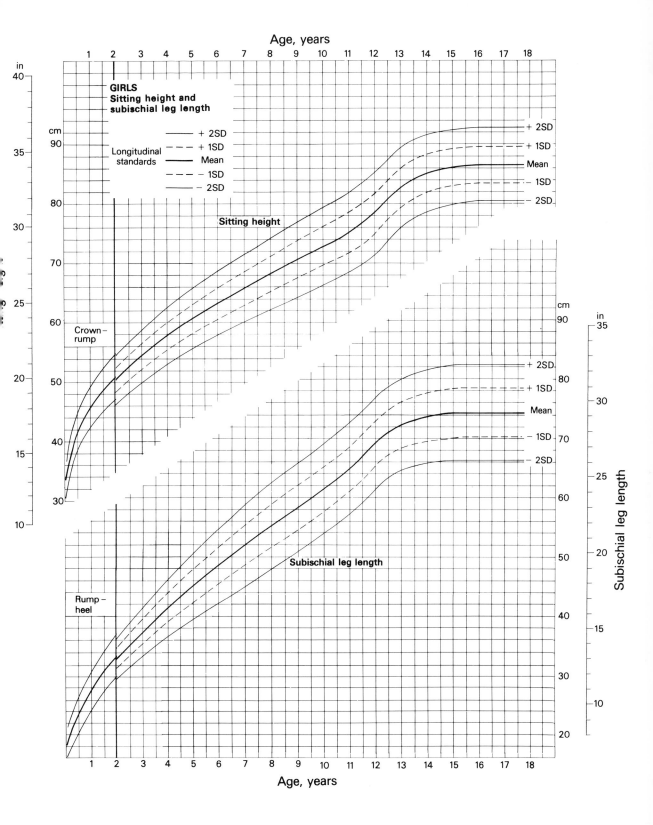

Figure 6.4 Centile chart relating sitting height and subischial leg length in girls (Castlemead Publications Chart No. LSHG49).

7: Biacromial and biiliac diameters

For measurement of biacromial diameter, the subject stands with shoulders relaxed and the measurer from behind applies the prongs of an anthropometer firmly to the outer edges of the acromial processes just above the shoulder joints. Similarly the biiliac diameter is measured from behind bringing the anthropometer arms on each side in firm contact with the outermost parts of the iliac crests (displacing any overlying fat).

Centile charts for these measurements are reproduced for boys and girls in Figures 7.1* to 7.4.

These measurements are seldom undertaken for clinical diagnostic purposes, but serially do demonstrate strikingly different patterns of growth through puberty in the two sexes. The biacromial diameter increases much more markedly in the male, but in both sexes the increase in biiliac diameter is quantitatively similar and therefore in the female greater in relation to increases in other body proportions. These diameters will reflect somatotypes which, in certain individuals, could account for discrepancies between weight and height centiles that might erroneously be attributed to fat.

*The figures in this chapter are based on unpublished data from Tanner J. M. and Whitehouse R. H.

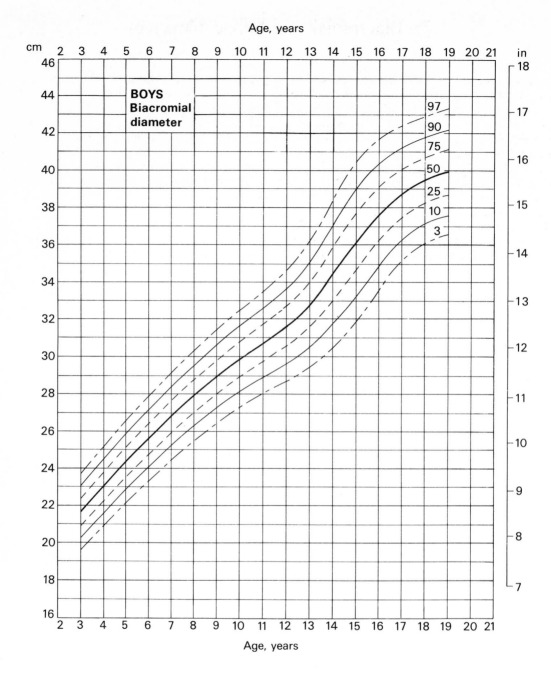

Figure 7.1 Centile chart for biacromial diameter for boys (Castlemead Publications Chart No. BCB34).

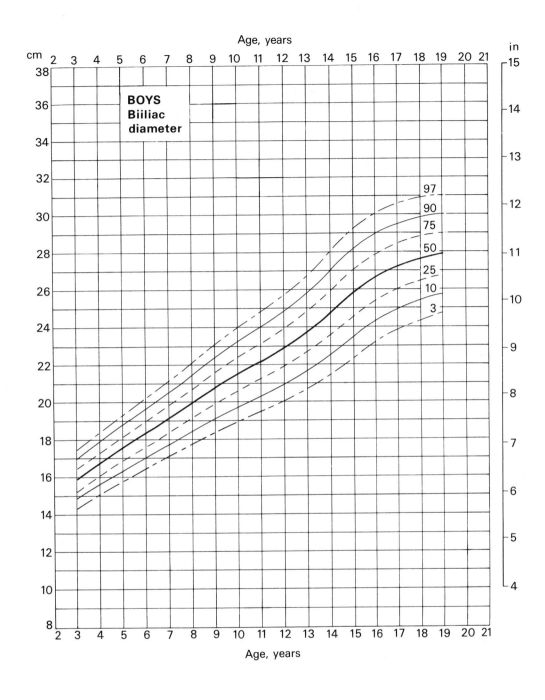

Figure 7.2 Centile chart for biiliac diameter for boys (Castlemead Publications Chart No. BIB36).

33

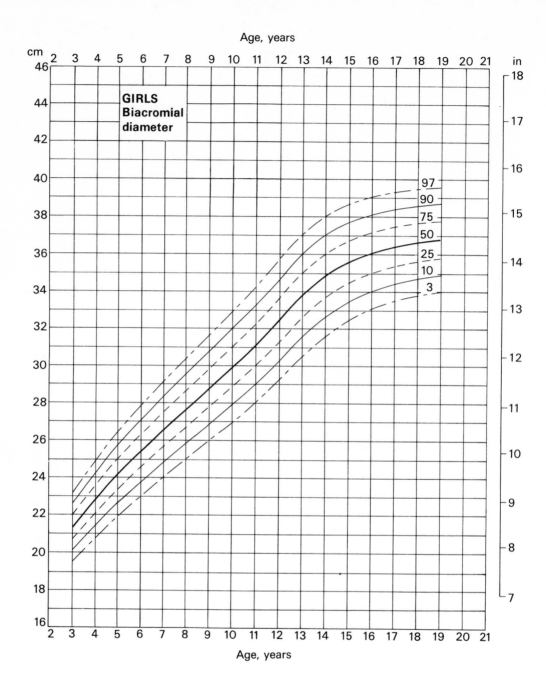

Figure 7.3 Centile chart for biacromial diameter for girls (Castlemead Publications Chart No. BCG35).

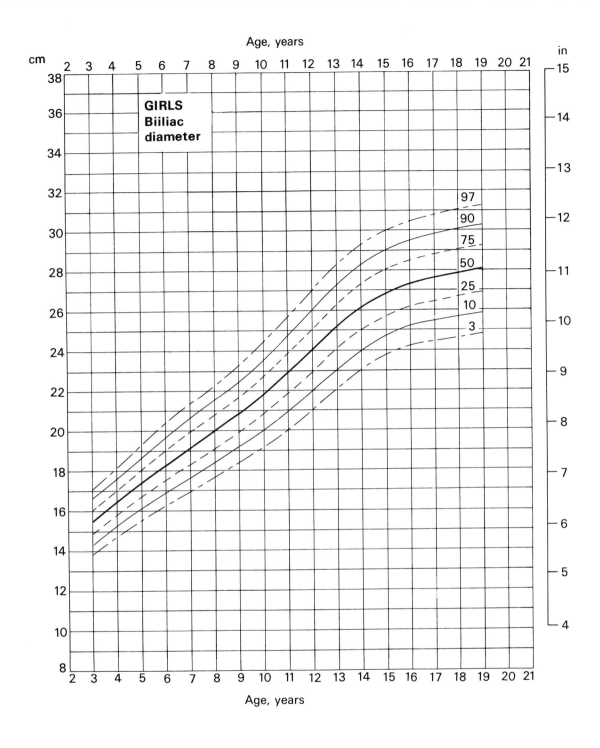

Figure 7.4 Centile chart for biiliac diameter for girls (Castlemead Publications Chart No. BIG37)

8: Skinfold measurements

Skinfold calipers are used for these measurements which show the thickness of subcutaneous tissue and reflect primarily fat. Several types of caliper are available. The Holtain and Harpenden varieties apply a constant pressure of 10 g/mm^2 over a measuring range of 0 mm to 48 mm and the measurements can be estimated to 0.1 mm. In neonates and young infants skinfold measurements can be obtained by similar techniques using the same instruments, but may prove more difficult as the baby is unlikely to remain still, and repeat measurements may be required to obtain a consistent reading.

Skinfolds can be measured at several sites, but the two most commonly used are the triceps and subscapular, which probably reflect best the body fat component as a whole.

The caliper is held with the right hand, and a fold of skin and subcutaneous tissue is lifted up from the underlying muscle between the thumb and index finger of the left hand. The jaws of the caliper are applied directly below to enclose this skinfold and the right hand is gently and completely relaxed for the jaws to apply their full constant pressure. The distance between the approximated jaws is read directly from the dial within a few seconds.

For comparative measurements it is advisable to use the same type of instrument and it is customary always to measure on the left side of the body and at precisely the same sites. Accuracy with experienced observers is of the order of ± 5%, but readings vary considerably with different measurers. Serial observations should preferably be undertaken by the same person.

The *triceps* skinfold is measured at a marked midpoint in the mid-posterior line of the left upper arm between the acromion and the olecranon processes with the arm extended and hanging loosely at the side.

The *subscapular* measurement is estimated, taking a vertical skinfold, directly below the angle of the left scapula.

Centile charts for boys and girls for triceps and subscapular skinfolds are reproduced in Figures 8.1* to 8.4 (Tanner and Whitehouse 1975). The centile distribution of these measurements is not linear, and is plotted on a logarithmic scale to which the distribution more closely approximates. In girls there is normally a steady increase in skinfold measurements from the age of about 6 years to maturity. In boys this increase is much less marked, and in fact shows a slight reduction in these measurements for a short period, approximately corresponding to the time of the pubertal growth spurt in height.

Skinfold measurements give an indication of the component of body weight that is fat. They aid in distinguishing those individuals whose weight is above the expected norm for their height because of increased lean body mass from those with excessive fat. These measurements are particularly valuable in following serially the progress of children in response to forms of treatment where expected weight gain through normal growth may tend to obscure changes resulting from treatment. Skinfold measurements are likely to increase on correction of malnutrition or treatment of thyrotoxicosis, and to fall in treating obesity or deficiencies of thyroid or growth hormone. At puberty, when changes in height and weight are expected to be marked, an indication of whether adipose tissue changes are within normal limits can be gained by observation of the centile positions of skinfold measurements.

---

*These figures are based on the standards originally presented by Tanner J. M. and Whitehouse R. H. in *Archives of Disease in Childhood*, **50**, 142, 1975 and are reproduced by permission of the authors and editors.

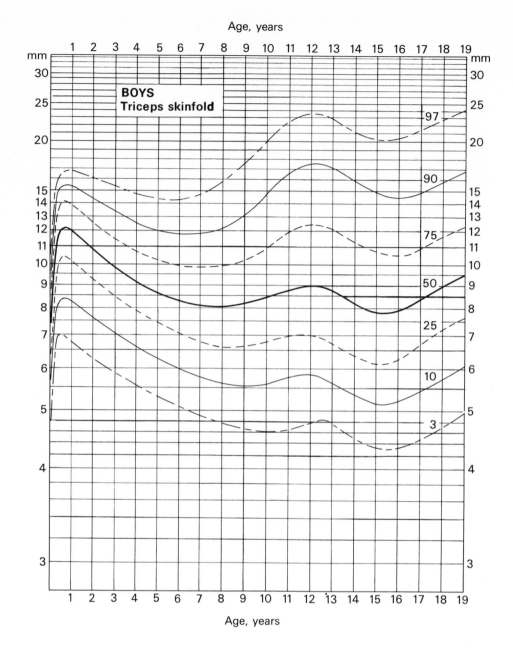

Figure 8.1 Centile chart for triceps skinfold for boys (Castlemead Publications Chart No. SKB45).

38

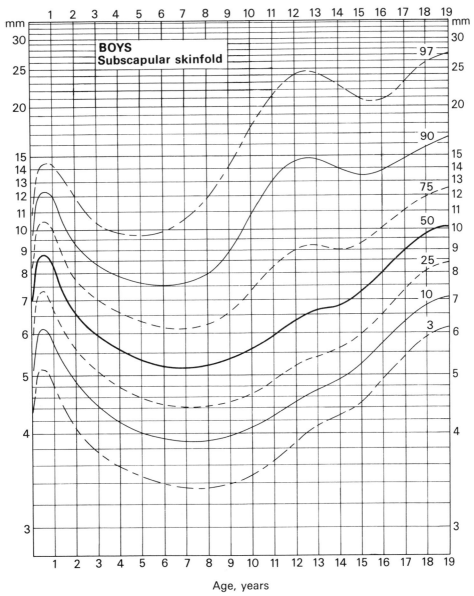

Figure 8.2 Centile chart for subscapular skinfold for boys (Castlemead Publications Chart No. SKB45).

39

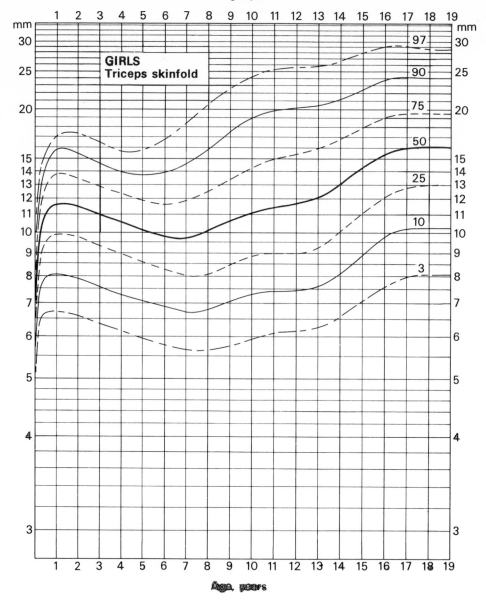

Figure 8.3 Centile chart for triceps skinfold for girls (Castlemead Publications Chart No. SKG46).

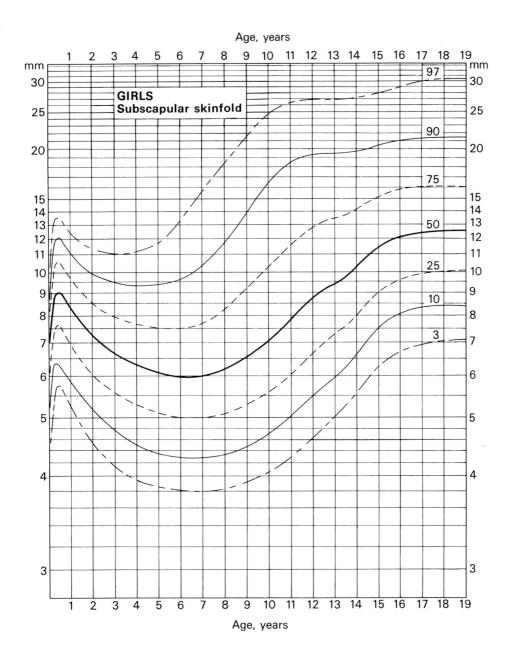

Figure 8.4 Centile chart for subscapular skinfold for girls (Castlemead Publications Chart No. SKG46).

9: Puberty

The stages of puberty are based on the descriptions of Tanner (1962) using standard ratings on a scale of 1 to 5. These are illustrated in Figures 9.1* and 9.2* for boys and girls respectively, which also show the centile distribution of the ages at which the various stages occur (2+ indicating that Stage 2 is reached but not yet Stage 3), as well as those for peak height velocity, testicular size in boys and menarche in girls. The centile values are shown in a similar way to that of Tanner and Whitehouse (1976) but the reverse of what might be expected. Thus the 97th centile represents the early age limit at which only 3% of children will show this feature and 97% remain to do so, and conversely the 3rd centile being the late end of the normal age range.

*These figures are based on the data of Tanner J. M. and Whitehouse R. H. in *Archives of Disease in Childhood*, **51**, 170, 1976 and are reproduced by permission of the authors and editors.

Boys: genital development

Stage 1 Preadolescent: the testes, scrotum and penis are of about the same size and proportions as in early childhood.

Stage 2 Enlargement of the scrotum and testes. The skin of the scrotum reddens and changes in texture. Little or no enlargement of the penis.

Stage 3 Lengthening of the penis. Further growth of the testes and scrotum.

Stage 4 Increase in breadth of the penis and development of the glans. The testes and scrotum are larger; the scrotum darkens.

Stage 5 Adult.

Boys: pubic hair

Stage 1 Preadolescent: no pubic hair.

Stage 2 Sparse growth of slightly pigmented downy hair chiefly at the base of the penis.

Stage 3 Hair darker, coarser and more curled, spreading sparsely over the junction of the pubes.

Stage 4 Hair adult in type, but covering a considerably smaller area than in the adult. No spread to the medial surface of the thighs.

Stage 5 Adult quantity and type with distribution of a horizontal pattern and spread to the medial surface of the thighs. Spread up linea alba is late and rated Stage 6.

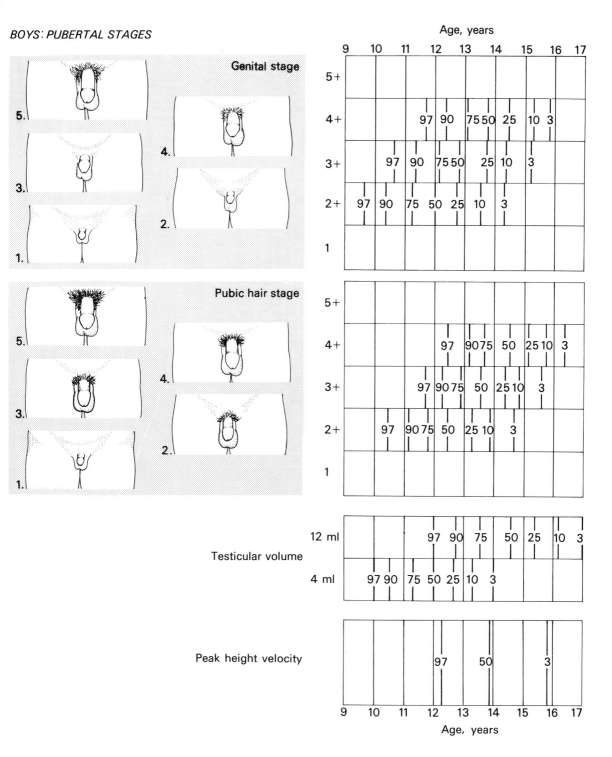

Figure 9.1 Stages of puberty in boys with centile distribution of ages.

45

Girls: breast development

Stage 1 Preadolescent: elevation of the papilla only.

Stage 2 Breast bud stage. Elevation of the breast and papilla as a small mound. Enlargement of the areola diameter.

Stage 3 Further enlargement and elevation of the breast and areola, with no separation of their contours.

Stage 4 Projection of the areola and papilla above the level of the breast.

Stage 5 Mature stage, projection of the papilla alone due to recession of the areola.

Girls: pubic hair

Stage 1 Preadolescent: no pubic hair.

Stage 2 Sparse growth of slightly pigmented downy hair chiefly along the labia.

Stage 3 Hair darker, coarser and more curled, spreading sparsely over the junction of the pubes.

Stage 4 Hair adult in type, but covering a considerably smaller area than in the adult. No spread to the medial surface of the thighs.

Stage 5 Adult quantity and type with distribution of a horizontal pattern and spread to the medial surface of the thighs. Spread up lines alba is late and rated Stage *6*.

GIRLS: PUBERTAL STAGES

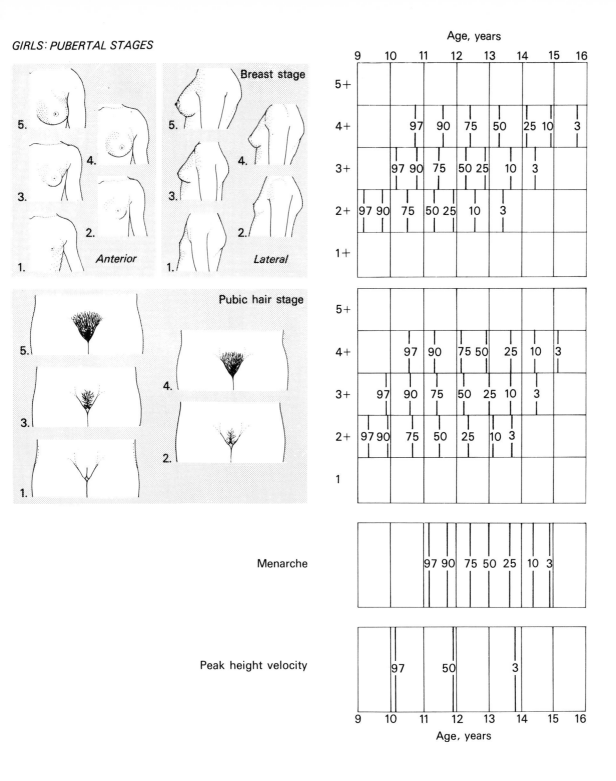

Figure 9.2 Stages of puberty in girls with centile distribution of ages.

47

Testicular size

This can be quantitatively assessed by comparison with a Prader orchidometer (Zachmann *et al.* 1974) either visually or by palpation. This is illustrated to scale in Figure 9.3, the number representing the volume of the testis in millilitres. Frequently the information required is merely whether the testis has grown to a larger than prepubertal size (1–3 ml) and a testis volume in excess of 5 ml is a good indication that puberty has started. Progress through puberty can be monitored according to testicular size, but variations in this in normal individuals at any stage of puberty are so great as to render such precise observations of little aid, and the adult testis varies between 12 and 25 ml. In Figure 9.1 only centiles for age of acquisition of two testicular volumes (4 ml and 12 ml) are shown (Tanner and Whitehouse, 1976).

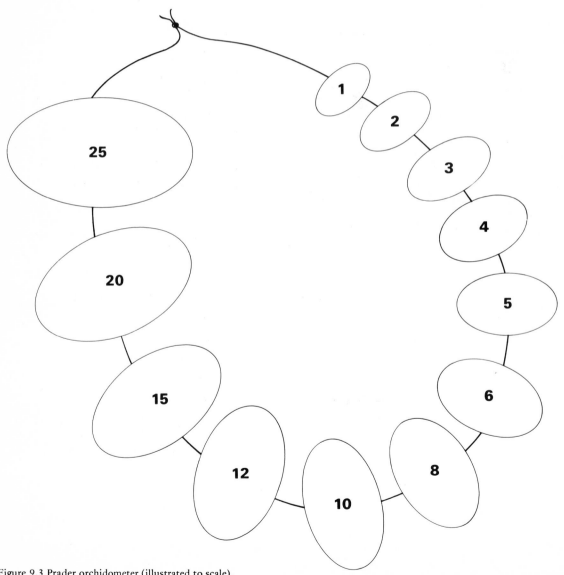

Figure 9.3 Prader orchidometer (illustrated to scale).

Breast development

It is not infrequent for one breast to develop earlier or faster than the other and staging would be accorded to that of the more advanced breast. Difficulties in breast rating may be experienced in obese children, though careful examination should distinguish between true breast tissue and adipose tissue. Single observations may occasionally make distinction between Stages 3 and 5 difficult, and a few girls never show Stage 4, passing straight from Stage 3 to 5, and a few others do not advance past Stage 4.

Relationship between pubertal changes

There is a great variation not only in the ages at which stages of puberty take place (as illustrated in Figures 9.1 and 9.2), but also in their duration and in the order in which they occur (Marshall and Tanner 1969 and 1970).

In *boys* the time taken for complete genital development averages about 3 years, but may be less than 2 or longer than 5. Full development of adult pubic hair is more rapid averaging about 1½ years, but may be less than 1 year or longer than 3. Pubic hair seldom appears before there are changes in external genitalia, and it may not commence before genital Stage 4. Peak height velocity is rarely achieved before genital Stage 4.

In *girls* development of the mature breast takes an average of 4 years, but may be as short as 1½ years or as long as 9 years; but as in boys, pubic hair development is more rapid, averaging 2½ years to reach the adult form, but may be less than 1½ years or longer than 3. About two-thirds of girls start to develop breasts before pubic hair growth commences, but the remainder show pubic hair first. Menarche usually occurs at breast stage 4, but in a quarter of girls it occurs in Stage 3 and in 10% not until Stage 5. The age of peak height velocity is relatively earlier in the course of puberty in girls than in boys and nearly always precedes the menarche, but by a rather variable interval which averages about a year.

The presence of some early changes of puberty (notably in boys increasing testicular size) provides evidence that normal progress through the stages of puberty is likely to follow forthwith. However some changes of puberty, such as development of pubic hair, may result from activity of androgens derived from the adrenal and need not, in either sex, be dependent on gonadal activity. Without evidence of gonadal activity (as indicated by growth of the gonads secondary to the stimulus of increased gonadotrophin secretion) development of isolated secondary sexual characteristics need not imply true puberty. Occasionally breast development alone may occur early (premature mammarche or thelarche) or pubic hair (premature pubarche or adrenarche) which may represent increased end organ responsiveness to relatively normal prepubertal hormonal levels.

Relationship of pubertal status to height

In view of the substantial contribution to ultimate height resulting from the pubertal growth spurt, interpretation of heights during the pubertal age range must be related to the stage of puberty attained. Peak height velocity in girls is relatively early in the sequence of pubertal change, whereas in boys it usually occurs late in the sequence, averaging 2 years later than girls. Moderate or minimal changes of puberty in boys probably indicate considerable remaining growth potential, whereas in girls advanced puberty, and notably an age past the menarche, suggest little remaining growth. The peak growth spurt is followed at a variable time by a cessation of growth due to bony fusion. The subject of prediction of adult height is considered in Chapter 11.

10: Skeletal maturity

Technique of assessment and merits of different methods

Various methods of estimating bone ages are available, and the choice depends on the degree of accuracy required. The bones of the wrist and hand are radiographically most useful for this purpose for the overall age range of the growing child. However, in infancy other centres are of greater value, and towards maturity X-ray of the knee indicates by the presence or absence of epiphyseal fusion whether significant residual growth in stature can be expected, although a little growth continues in the spine after it is completed in the limbs.

1. Ages of appearance of ossific centres

For everyday clinical purposes requiring only single observations to exclude major deviations from the normal, this simple system is adequate. Figure 10.1 illustrates for boys and girls the mean age of appearance and fusion of the bony centres of the wrist and hand. Figure 10.2 shows the age of appearance of centres in various other sites that are most likely to be useful and these are listed in tabular form in Figure 10.3 for boys and girls. This technique is not, however, precise enough for accurate observations, particularly when these are undertaken serially.

2. Atlas of Pyle, Waterhouse and Greulich (1971)

This system is based on a series of 25 X-rays of wrists and hands of children of ages ranging from birth to maturity, each picture being designated an age to which it most closely corresponds within a normal population. This population is, however, an upperclass American one and does not correspond to the cross section of British children, or children of other nationalities. A simple adjustment can, however, be made to the estimates based on this system to correct for the British population, and this is shown graphically in Figures 10.4 and 10.5 for boys and girls (Buckler 1977). The discrepancy may be considerable (over 18 months) at certain ages.

This method, though more accurate than 1, is still approximate, being based primarily on the appearance of the carpal centres, which do not necessarily show a consistent order or pattern, and matching with these standards may not always be easy. Observations of the long bones of the hand are seldom included when using this technique, but if they are, discrepancies may be even more marked as the relationship between the development of round bone and long bone centres is very variable.

Nevertheless, this system is quick and usually simple and, for many purposes not requiring great accuracy, is adequate, provided a correction is made for a British (or other) population. It is essential to match the bone standards appropriately for sex, as girls are always markedly advanced in their bony development compared with boys. This is demonstrated in Figure 10.1 which shows the ages in boys and girls for which the same levels of skeletal maturity would correspond. This figure also illustrates the radiological appearances of hands corresponding to various ages (as indicated in the boxes) for average British boys and girls.

An alternative atlas of skeletal age has recently been introduced from the Netherlands (DeRoo and Schröder 1976). Based presumably on European standards, it has much to recommend it. However, the bone ages illustrated are still somewhat advanced compared with the British standards of Tanner and Whitehouse.

3. Tanner and Whitehouse System

This is a more accurate technique based on radiographs of hands and wrists of middle class British boys and girls. The method involves the designation of a score for the state of development of 20 bones in the wrist and hand. The original system (TW1) (Tanner et al. 1962), has recently been modified (TW2) (Tanner et al. 1975a), so that maturity scores can be derived from 7 carpal centres alone (TW2 carpal), or from the centres of the lower radial and ulnar epiphyses and of selected digits totalling 13 bones (TW2 RUS), as well as combining them in the 20-bone system (TW2 20-bone). The carpal bones alone give little precise data in infancy and later adolescence, but are of greater value in the intervening periods where changes are more striking. The long bones, on the other hand, give greater information over these extreme ages of childhood, and the full TW2 20-bone method gives an accurate assessment over the whole range of childhood. For each centre or bone a score is designated appropriate for its level of development, and the total of these scores gives a value ('skeletal maturity score') for which a skeletal age can be read directly from tables. Charts for these data, showing the centile distributions of the skeletal maturity scores with age, are available (see Appendix, p. 100).

This technique is time consuming, but takes account of variations in progress of maturation of the individual bones, and so is much more precise. It is however only feasible for regular use in specialised growth centres or for those undertaking research projects.

51

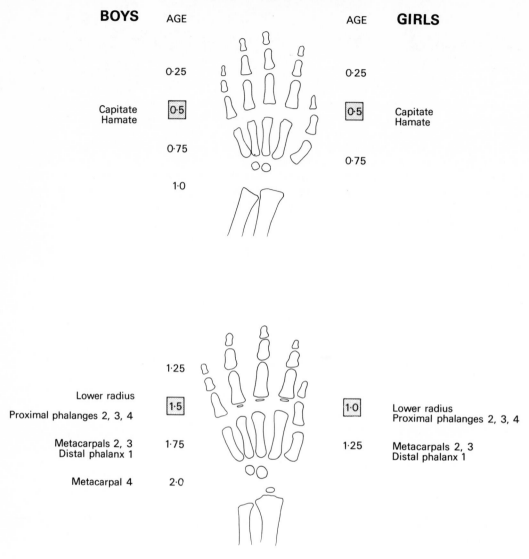

Average age of appearance of centres

BOYS   AGE   AGE   **GIRLS**

0·25   0·25

Capitate Hamate   0·5   0·5   Capitate Hamate

0·75   0·75

1·0

1·25

Lower radius
Proximal phalanges 2, 3, 4   1·5   1·0   Lower radius
Proximal phalanges 2, 3, 4

Metacarpals 2, 3
Distal phalanx 1   1·75   1·25   Metacarpals 2, 3
Distal phalanx 1

Metacarpal 4   2·0

Figure 10.1 Mean age of appearance and fusion of the ossific centres of the wrist and hand for British boys and girls. The illustrations shown correspond to the boxed ages.

52

Average age of appearance of centres

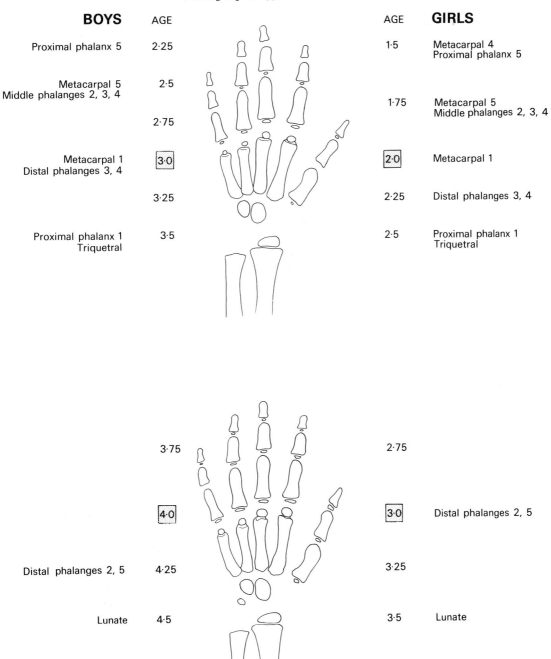

BOYS	AGE		AGE	GIRLS
Proximal phalanx 5	2·25		1·5	Metacarpal 4 Proximal phalanx 5
Metacarpal 5 Middle phalanges 2, 3, 4	2·5			
	2·75		1·75	Metacarpal 5 Middle phalanges 2, 3, 4
Metacarpal 1 Distal phalanges 3, 4	3·0		2·0	Metacarpal 1
	3·25		2·25	Distal phalanges 3, 4
Proximal phalanx 1 Triquetral	3·5		2·5	Proximal phalanx 1 Triquetral
	3·75		2·75	
	4·0		3·0	Distal phalanges 2, 5
Distal phalanges 2, 5	4·25		3·25	
Lunate	4·5		3·5	Lunate

Figure 10.1 *continued*

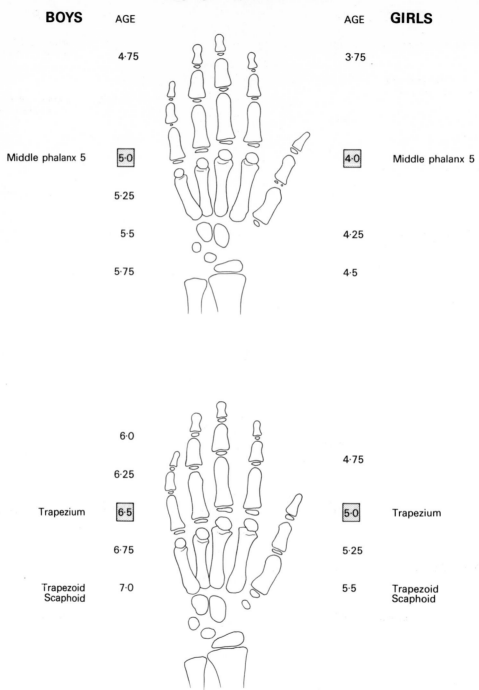

Average age of appearance of centres

BOYS   AGE   AGE   GIRLS

4·75   3·75

Middle phalanx 5   5·0   4·0   Middle phalanx 5

5·25

5·5   4·25

5·75   4·5

6·0   4·75

6·25

Trapezium   6·5   5·0   Trapezium

6·75   5·25

Trapezoid   7·0   5·5   Trapezoid
Scaphoid   Scaphoid

Figure 10.1 Mean age of appearance and fusion of the ossific centres of the wrist and hand for British boys and girls. The illustrations shown correspond to the boxed ages.

Average age of appearance of centres

BOYS AGE

7·25

AGE **GIRLS**

5·75

Lower ulna 7·5

6·0 Lower ulna

7·75

6·25

8·0

6·5

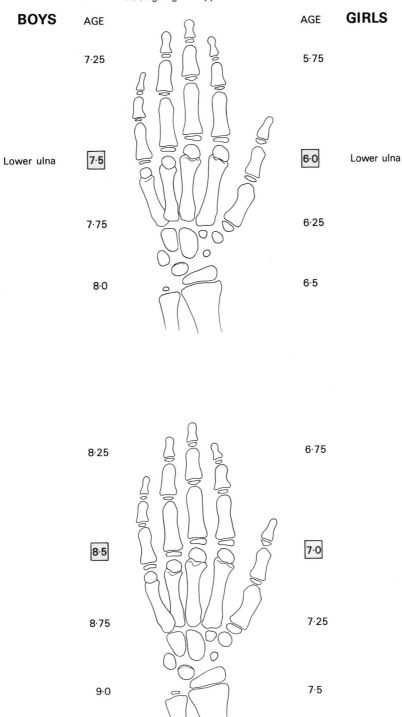

8·25

6·75

8·5

7·0

8·75

7·25

9·0

7·5

Figure 10.1 *continued*

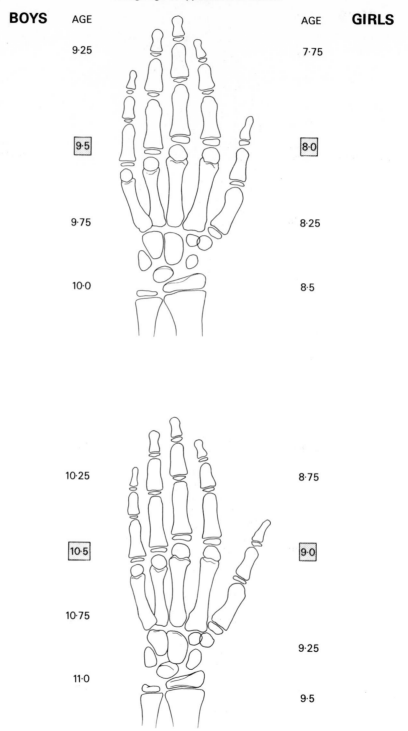

Average age of appearance of centres

BOYS   AGE   AGE   GIRLS

9·25   7·75

9·5   8·0

9·75   8·25

10·0   8·5

10·25   8·75

10·5   9·0

10·75   9·25

11·0   9·5

Figure 10.1 Mean age of appearance and fusion of the ossific centres of the wrist and hand for British boys and girls. The illustrations shown correspond to the boxed ages.

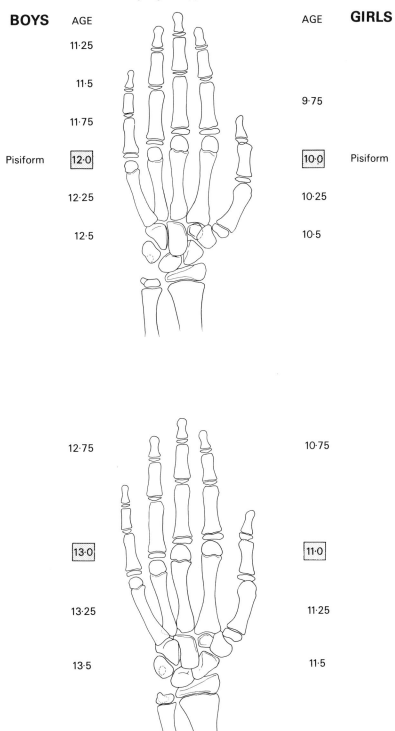

BOYS AGE

11·25

11·5

11·75

Pisiform 12·0

12·25

12·5

12·75

13·0

13·25

13·5

AGE **GIRLS**

9·75

10·0 Pisiform

10·25

10·5

10·75

11·0

11·25

11·5

Figure 10.1 *continued*

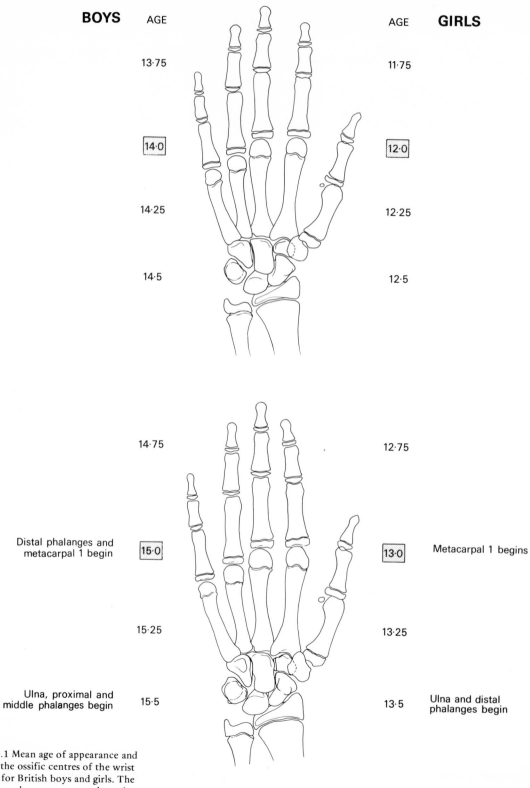

BOYS   AGE

13·75

14·0

14·25

14·5

14·75

Distal phalanges and
metacarpal 1 begin   15·0

15·25

Ulna, proximal and
middle phalanges begin   15·5

AGE   **GIRLS**

11·75

12·0

12·25

12·5

12·75

13·0   Metacarpal 1 begins

13·25

13·5   Ulna and distal
phalanges begin

Figure 10.1 Mean age of appearance and
fusion of the ossific centres of the wrist
and hand for British boys and girls. The
illustrations shown correspond to the
boxed ages.

Average age of fusion of centres

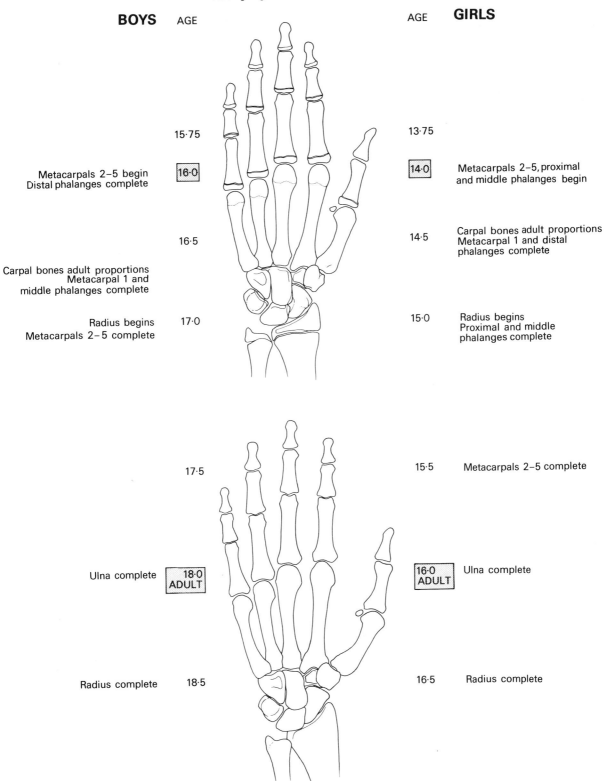

BOYS AGE

	15·75
Metacarpals 2–5 begin Distal phalanges complete	**16·0**
	16·5
Carpal bones adult proportions Metacarpal 1 and middle phalanges complete	
Radius begins Metacarpals 2–5 complete	17·0
	17·5
Ulna complete	**18·0 ADULT**
Radius complete	18·5

AGE GIRLS

13·75	
14·0	Metacarpals 2–5, proximal and middle phalanges begin
14·5	Carpal bones adult proportions Metacarpal 1 and distal phalanges complete
15·0	Radius begins Proximal and middle phalanges complete
15·5	Metacarpals 2–5 complete
16·0 ADULT	Ulna complete
16·5	Radius complete

Figure 10.1 *continued*

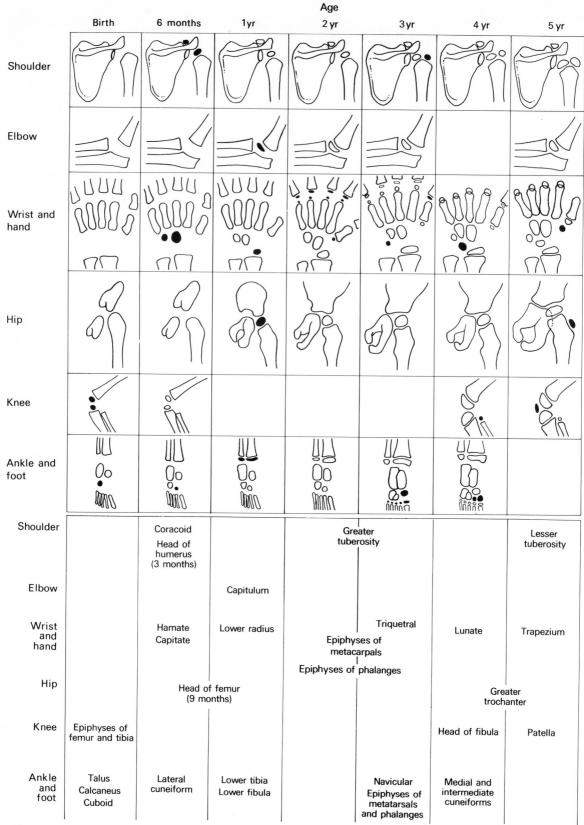

Figure 10.2 Mean ages of appearance of ossific centres of the bones of the upper and lower limbs. New centres of ossification appearing at each stage are shown in black.

Age

	6 yr	7 yr	8 yr	9 yr	10 yr	11 yr	12–13 yr
Shoulder							
Elbow							
Wrist and hand							
Hip							
Knee							
Ankle and foot							

	6 yr	7 yr	8 yr	9 yr	10 yr	11 yr	12–13 yr
Shoulder	Union of head and greater tuberosity						
Elbow	Head of radius	Medial epicondyle			Medial trochlea	Olecranon	Lateral epicondyle
Wrist and hand	Trapezoid Scaphoid	Lower ulna			Pisiform		
Hip				Union of ischium and pubis	Lesser trochanter		
Knee						Tibial tuberosity sometimes separate centre	
Ankle and foot				Epiphysis of calcaneus			

61

		Boys	Girls
ARM			
Scapula	Coracoid	Birth–1 yr	Birth–1 yr
Humerus	Head	Birth or soon after	Birth or soon after
	Greater tuberosity	3 yr	2 yr
	Lesser tuberosity	5 yr	5 yr
	Medial epicondyle	8–9 yr	5–6 yr
	Capitulum and lateral trochlea	1–1½ yr	1–1½ yr
	Medial trochlea	10 yr	10 yr
	Lateral epicondyle	14 yr	14 yr
Ulna	Olecranon	11 yr	11 yr
	Distal	7–8 yr	6–7 yr
Radius	Head	6–7 yr	5–6 yr
	Distal	1–1½ yr	1 yr
Hand		See Fig. 10.1	See Fig. 10.1
LEG			
Femur	Head	½–1 yr	½–1 yr
	Greater trochanter	5 yr	4 yr
	Lesser trochanter	9–11 yr	9–11 yr
	Distal epiphysis	Birth	Birth
Patella		4–5 yr	4–5 yr
Tibia	Proximal	Birth	Birth
	Distal	½–1 yr	½–1 yr
Fibula	Proximal	3–4 yr	3 yr
	Distal	1 yr	1 yr
Foot	Talus	Birth	Birth
	Calcaneus	Birth	Birth
	Epiphysis of Calcaneus	10 yr	8 yr
	Cuboid	Birth	Birth
	Lateral cuneiform	0–1 yr	0–1 yr
	Intermediate cuneiform	4 yr	3 yr
	Medial cuneiform	4 yr	3 yr
	Navicular	2–3 yr	2–3 yr
	Metatarsals: secondary centres base of 1, head of others	3 yr	2 yr
	Phalanges: secondary centres	3 yr	2 yr

Figure 10.3 Mean ages of appearance of ossific centres of the bones of the upper and lower limbs of boys and girls.

Value and interpretation of skeletal ages

Diagnostic

A knowledge of the degree of advancement or delay in bone age and its relationship to height age is of considerable value in diagnosing conditions in childhood related to abnormal patterns of growth and sexual development. This information is increased by observations of the trend in bone age over the course of time. However, by far the commonest cause of moderate retardation or advancement of skeletal age is physiological variation.

Prognostic

Bone age may indicate the amount of remaining growth potential in a child, and in this respect is a better index than chronological age. This relationship is only approximate, however, and at pubertal ages is not well related to the stage of puberty except to the menarche. Where bone age is retarded for a pathological cause as distinct from a physiological variant, the growth potential that is indicated by bone age will only be forthcoming if the condition is treatable and treated. Conversely, with pathologically advanced bone age, particularly if height age is advanced less than skeletal age, growth potential is likely to be reduced, with ultimate short stature.

In monitoring treatment

The relationship between chronological age, height age and skeletal age, observed serially, is a useful aid in evaluating treatment, particularly of endocrine disorders of growth.

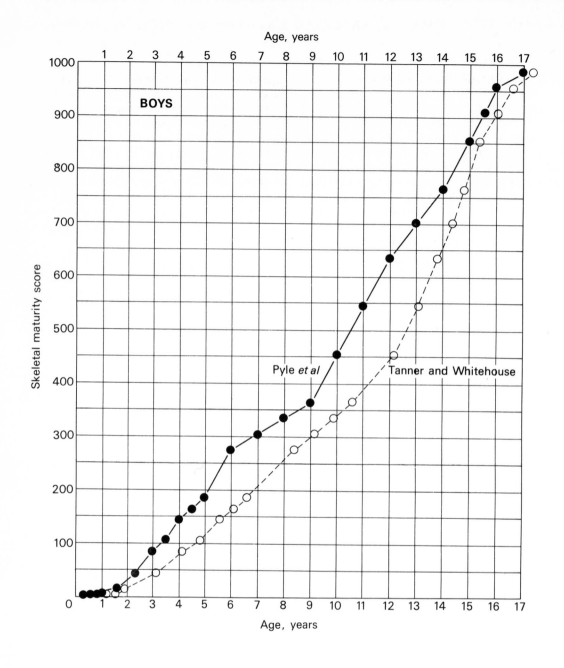

Figure 10.4 Comparison of skeletal age assessments by the methods of Pyle *et al.* (1971), and Tanner *et al.* (1975a) for boys.

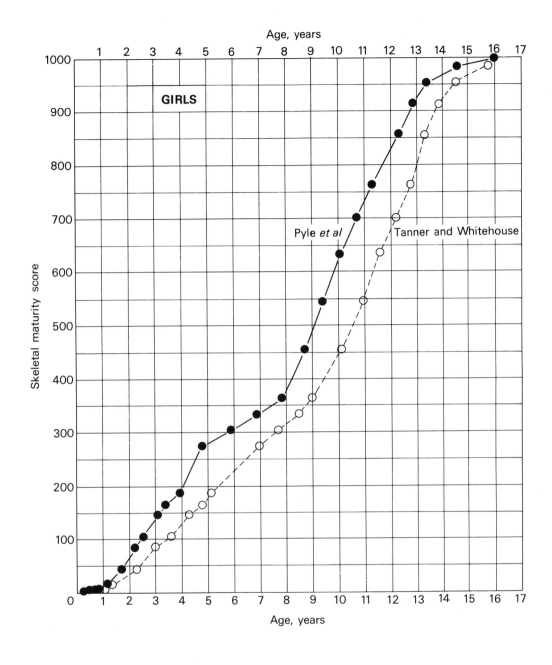

Figure 10.5 Comparison of skeletal age assessments by the methods of Pyle *et al.* (1971), and Tanner *et al.* (1975a) for girls.

11: Prediction of adult height

In predicting adult height, not only is the actual height of the child at a particular age of importance, but also the skeletal maturity, pubertal status and parental heights.

Tanner *et al.* (1975b) have developed an equation for predicting adult height (H_A) depending on values for height, chronological age and skeletal age:

H_A = [Height (cm) $\times$ Value A]

minus [Chronological age (yr) $\times$ Value B]

minus [Skeletal age (yr) $\times$ Value C]

plus [Constant value D]

The values A, B, C and D are given for appropriate age ranges in Figures 11.1* and 11.2* for boys and girls, with variants for girls between 11 and 15 years depending on whether they are pre- or post-menarcheal. The bone age estimation in the original equation was based on the TW2 RUS score (13 long bones; Tanner *et al.* 1975b see p.48) but the difference resulting from the use of the full TW2 20 bone score or carpal bone score is very small. The tables also give standard deviation (S.D.) values. The adult height of 95% of subjects will fall within 2 S.D. of the *predicted* adult height. This range will be considerably narrower than the 95% height range of the total adult population, which is ± 12.5 cm for males and ± 11.5 cm for females. The S.D. values become progressively smaller and the predictions more accurate in older children, and in girls after the menarche. A further correction can be made for parental height, but it is doubtful whether the resulting improvement in the accuracy of the prediction is statistically significant.

*Based on the data of Tanner J. M. *et al.* (1975) *Archives of Disease in Childhood*, **50**, 14, and reproduced by permission of the authors and editors.

Age (yr)	Value A (Height)	Value B (Chronological age)	Value C (Bone age (RUS))	Value D Constant	Residual S.D. (cm)	r
4, 5, 6, 7 +	1.20	−7.3	0	82	4.0	0.84
8.0−	1.22	−7.2	−0.4	82	3.6	0.89
8.5−	1.23	−7.0	−0.7	82		
9.0−	1.22	−6.8	−0.8	82	3.6	0.89
9.5−	1.21	−6.5	−0.8	82		
10.0−	1.20	−6.2	−1.0	83	3.6	0.89
10.5−	1.19	−5.9	−1.2	84		
11.0−	1.16	−5.5	−1.6	89	3.5	0.89
11.5−	1.13	−5.1	−2.0	94		
12.0−	1.08	−4.2	−2.6	98	3.5	0.88
12.5−	1.03	−3.4	−3.2	103		
13.0−	0.98	−2.6	−3.8	108	3.1	0.89
13.5−	0.94	−1.9	−4.4	113		
14.0−	0.90	−1.4	−4.5	114	2.9	0.90
14.5−	0.87	−1.0	−4.6	114		
15.0−	0.84	−0.8	−3.8	104	2.5	0.92
15.5−	0.82	−0.6	−3.1	94		
16.0−	0.88	−0.4	−2.4	71	2.0	0.96
16.5−	0.94	−0.3	−1.8	48		
17.0−	0.96	−0.2	−1.2	34	0.8	0.99
17.5−	0.98	−0.1	−0.7	19		

Figure 11.1 Table for prediction of adult height for boys.

Age (yr)	Value A (Height)	Value B (Chronological age)	Value C (Bone age (RUS))	Value D Constant	Residual S.D. (cm)	r
4, 5 +	0.95	− 6.5	0	93	3.5	0.85
6.0−	0.95	− 6.0	− 0.4	93 ⎫	3.0	0.86
6.5−	0.95	− 5.5	− 0.8	93 ⎭		
7.0−	0.94	− 5.1	− 1.0	94 ⎫	3.2	0.85
7.5−	0.93	− 4.7	− 1.1	94 ⎭		
8.0−	0.92	− 4.4	− 1.5	95 ⎫	2.9	0.89
8.5−	0.92	− 4.0	− 1.9	96 ⎭		
9.0−	0.92	− 3.8	− 2.3	99 ⎫	2.8	0.85
9.5−	0.91	− 3.6	− 2.7	102 ⎭		
10.0−	0.89	− 3.2	− 3.2	106 ⎫	2.9	0.85
10.5−	0.87	− 2.7	− 3.6	109 ⎭		
Premenarcheal						
11.0−	0.83	− 2.6	− 3.6	114 ⎫	2.9	0.82
11.5−	0.82	− 2.5	− 3.6	115 ⎭		
12.0−	0.83	− 2.4	− 3.4	111 ⎫	2.7	0.87
12.5−	0.83	− 2.3	− 3.3	108 ⎭		
13.0−	0.85	− 2.0	− 3.1	98 ⎫	2.2	0.92
13.5−	0.87	− 1.8	− 3.0	90 ⎭		
14.0−	0.91	− 1.6	− 2.8	79 ⎫	1.2	0.94
14.5−	0.95	− 1.4	− 2.5	67 ⎭		
Postmenarcheal						
11.0−	0.87	− 2.3	− 3.3	100 ⎫	2.6*	0.87*
11.5−	0.89	− 1.9	− 3.3	91 ⎭		
12.0−	0.91	− 1.4	− 3.2	82 ⎫	2.1	0.89
12.5−	0.93	− 1.0	− 2.7	67 ⎭		
13.0−	0.95	− 0.9	− 2.2	55 ⎫	1.6	0.94
13.5−	0.96	− 0.9	− 1.8	48 ⎭		
14.0−	0.96	− 0.8	− 1.4	40 ⎫	1.2	0.97
14.5−	0.97	− 0.8	− 1.3	37 ⎭		
All girls						
15.0−	0.98	− 0.6	− 1.1	30 ⎫	0.8	0.99
15.5−	0.99	− 0.4	− 0.7	20 ⎭		

*Values estimated.

Figure 11.2 Table for prediction of adult height for girls.

12: Head circumference

Technique of measurement

Head circumference should represent the maximum measurement around the head in the horizontal plane. It is best performed using a tape measure made of a non-stretch material, preferably a narrow pliable steel measure. For infants, an assistant may be required to hold the head and ensure correct positioning of the tape.

Recording

There are considerable differences in the centile values for head circumference presented in charts from different sources, related presumably to the populations from which they were derived. The centile charts included here are considered best for representation of the typical British population. Figures 12.1* and 12.3* can be used up to the age of 2 years (Gairdner and Pearson 1971). They show the 10th, 50th and 90th centiles and include a correction for duration of gestation (see Chapter 15). In babies born preterm the difference between the real birth date and the expected date of delivery is subtracted from the infants actual age in determining where to plot the measurements. The charts can also be used for weight and length recordings and so provide a means of comparing these values with head circumference. From the age of 2 years until maturity the centile charts in Figures 12.2† and 12.4† can be used.

Interpretation

The marked variations that occur in head shape, particularly in the immediate neonatal period, indicate that head circumference measurements alone may not necessarily give an accurate reflection of skull capacity. Several factors should be considered in an interpretation of head circumference measurements.

(a) Serial measurements. These are usually more informative than single ones in indicating pathology. A head circumference which adheres to the same centile position as time progresses is more likely to be normal than one which is accelerating or falling away from the lines.

(b) Relation to body size. Head size that appears abnormal may be appropriate when related to length and weight centiles. A gross discrepancy between these centile values makes pathology more likely. Heads may, however, be relatively large in children suffering from malnutrition.

(c) Features of sutures and fontanelles. In many conditions where head size is abnormal, an underlying cause may also result in abnormalities in size and tension of fontanelles and width of sutures.

(d) Correction for gestational age. This should be included as already indicated.

(e) Familial factors. Small, large or strangely shaped heads which do not represent any significant pathology may be explained on a familial basis by observations of the sizes and shapes of the heads of parents and siblings.

*Based on standards presented by Gairdner D. and Pearson J. (1971) *Archives of Disease in Childhood*, 46, 783, and reproduced by permission of the authors and editors.
†Standards derived by Tanner and Whitehouse and reproduced by their permission, based on two sets of comparable data described in Falkner F. (1958) *Archives of Disease in Childhood*, 33, 1, and the Oxford Child Health Survey reported by Westropp C. K. and Barber C. R. (1956) *Journal of Neurology, Neurosurgery and Psychiatry*, 19, 52.

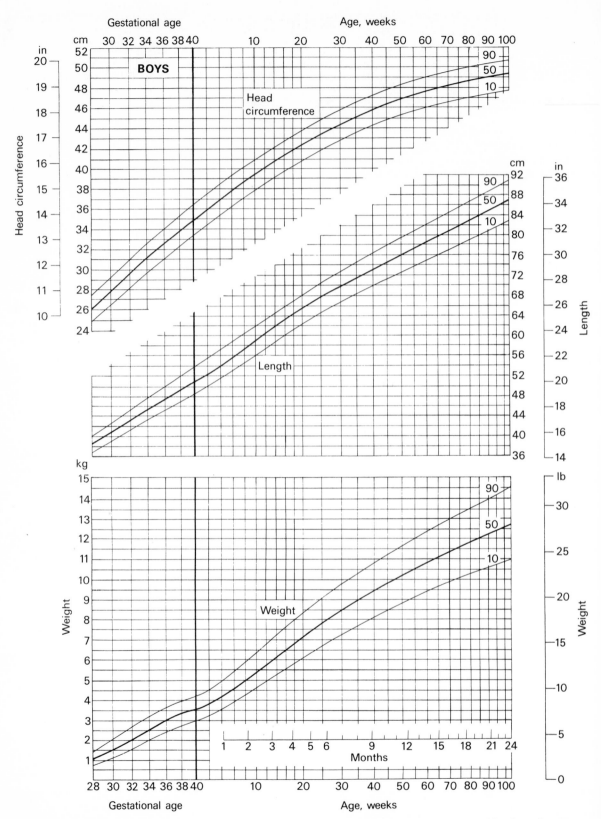

Figure 12.1 Head circumference, length and weight centile chart for boys aged 0–2 years (Castlemead Publications Chart No. GPB).

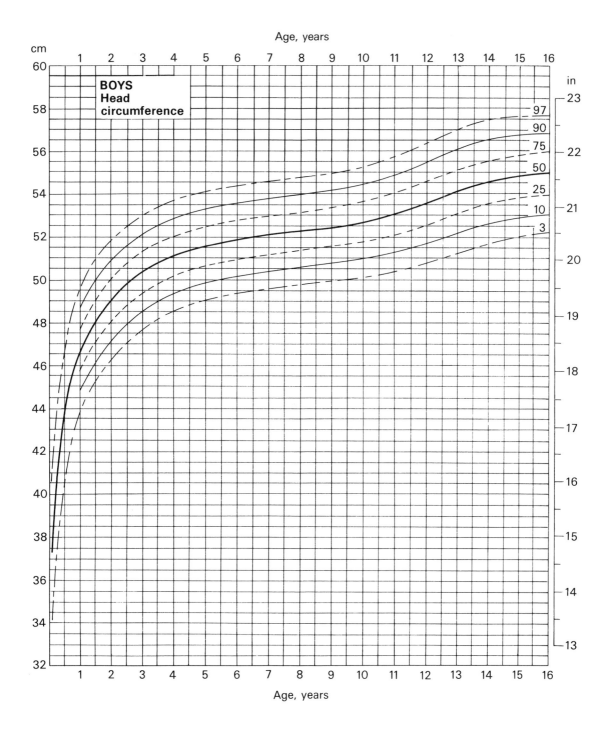

Figure 12.2 Head circumference centile chart for boys aged 0–16 years (Castlemead Publications Chart No. HCB18).

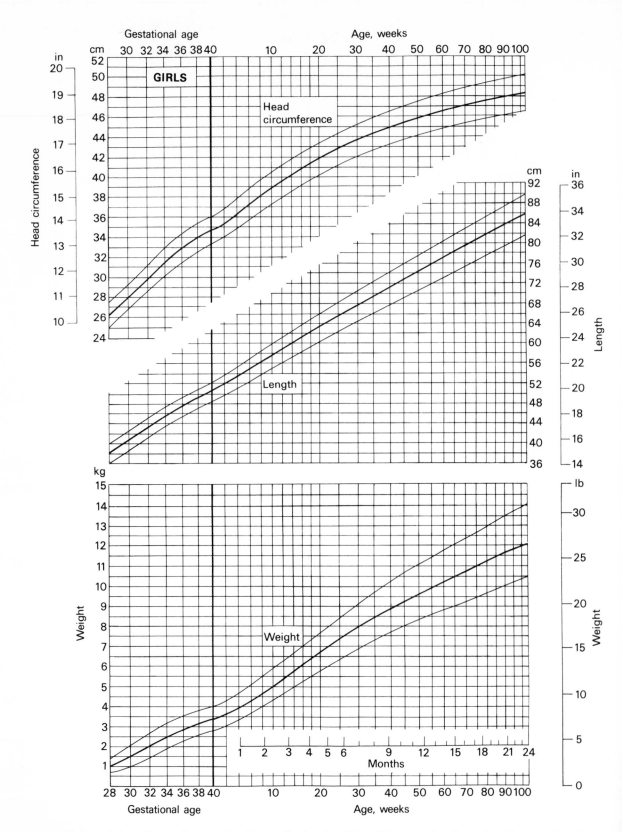

Figure 12.3 Head circumference, length and weight centile chart for girls aged 0–2 years (Castlemead Publications Chart No. GPG).

72

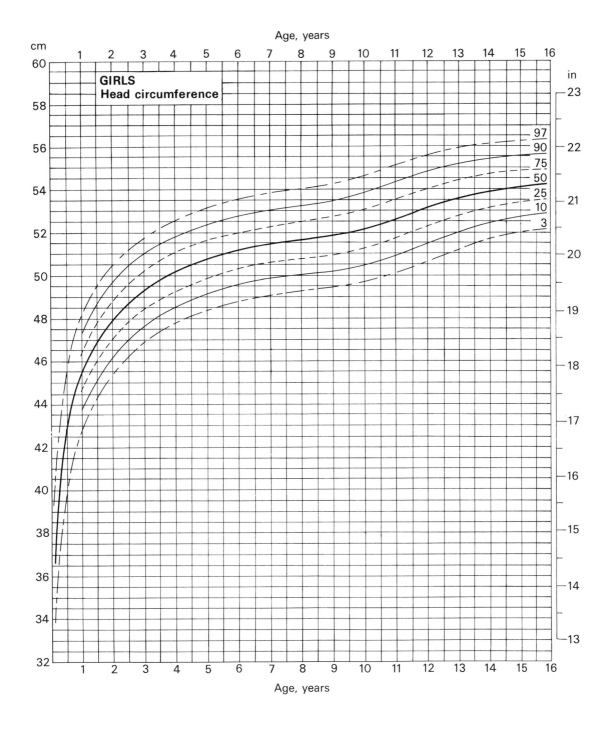

Figure 12.4 Head circumference centile chart for girls aged 0–16 years (Castlemead Publications Chart No. HCG19).

13: Dental development

Primary teeth

Primary (deciduous) teeth are often identified by capital letters:

A = central incisor
B = lateral incisor
C = canine
D = first molar
E = second molar.

The full primary dentition may be depicted thus:

	Right		Left	
	Right		Left	
Upper	E D C B A		A B C D E	
Lower	E D C B A		A B C D E	

Primary teeth commence to calcify at about 3–4 months intra-uterine life and usually erupt at ages between 6 months and 24 months. The sequence of eruption is A B D C E with the lower teeth usually erupting slightly in advance of the upper teeth. Thus the first teeth to erupt are the lower central incisors or $\overline{A|A}$, and the last teeth to erupt are the upper second molars or E | E.

The number of teeth an infant would be expected to have at a particular age is shown in Figure 13.1 with 10th, 50th and 90th centile distributions (Harvey and Parkinson 1977). Though there is considerable variation in the eruption times of deciduous teeth, the duration of the eruption period is relatively constant, being about 22 months.

Among variations which influence age and pattern of eruption of teeth in normal children are racial factors, familial factors and body size. The teeth of larger infants erupt earlier than those of smaller ones. It sometimes happens that $\overline{A|A}$ or just $\overline{A|}$ or $\overline{|A}$ are present at birth. These teeth, called neonatal teeth, have no roots and have a very loose attachment to the mucosa. Because these teeth may be dislodged during feeding, it is wise to remove them.

Normally the roots of primary teeth continue to develop for 2 years after tooth eruption, but 3 years following eruption the roots normally begin to be resorbed due to pressure from succeeding secondary teeth. When all the root or roots (molars have more than one root) of a tooth have been resorbed, the crown is shed and the succeeding secondary tooth takes its place. In general, primary teeth are shed in the order in which they erupt, i.e. A B D C E, with lowers preceding uppers. Thus the first teeth to be shed are usually $\overline{A|A}$, and the last teeth to be shed are E | E.

Secondary teeth

There are normally 32 secondary teeth, 8 in each quadrant of the mouth.

The secondary dentition is often depicted by Arabic numerals:

1 central incisor
2 lateral incisor
3 canine
4 first premolar
5 second premolar
6 first molar
7 second molar
8 third molar or wisdom tooth.

	Right		Left	
	Right		Left	
Upper	8 7 6 5 4 3 2 1		1 2 3 4 5 6 7 8	
Lower	8 7 6 5 4 3 2 1		1 2 3 4 5 6 7 8	

The molar teeth 6, 7 and 8, do not succeed primary teeth, but those numbered 1, 2, 3, 4, and 5 do. Thus 1 replaces A, 2 replaces B, 3 replaces C, 4 replaces D and 5 replaces E.

The first secondary tooth to erupt is the first permanent molar (No. 6) which normally erupts at about 6 years of age. The second molar (No. 7) erupts at about 12 years of age, and the third molar (wisdom tooth, No. 8) erupts at about 18 years of age. The normal order of eruption according to tooth number is 6, 1, 2, 3, 4, 5, 7, 8, with the lowers erupting just in advance of the uppers. Figure 13.2 indicates the average age of eruption of permanent teeth and is based on a recent cross-sectional study of 845 York schoolboys and girls aged between 5 and 15 years (Jackson & Fairpo 1976). These data have also been presented in Figure 13.3 to show the number of teeth erupted at various ages with the 10th, 50th and 90th centiles. There is considerable variation in the age of tooth eruption and these figures only serve as a guideline being based on a relatively small series and without any separation according to sex.

There is an approximate correlation between skeletal age and the eruption of teeth. In those children with a skeletal age greater than their chronological age, teeth erupt earlier, and in those with a retarded skeletal age the opposite occurs. As girls mature more quickly than boys, their teeth erupt earlier (by approximately 6 months).

There are several factors that interfere with the normal eruption of secondary teeth. In some children there is an incompatibility between the size of jaws and the size of teeth. When the jaws are too small some teeth cannot find enough room to erupt and remain impacted in the bone. Third molars (wisdom teeth) are notorious in their liability to be impacted. Occasionally there are extra teeth, most commonly seen in the upper incisor region. These extra teeth can impede and deflect the eruption of neighbouring teeth.

Certain teeth may be congenitally absent, the commonest being the upper lateral incisors, the lower second premolars, and the third molars.

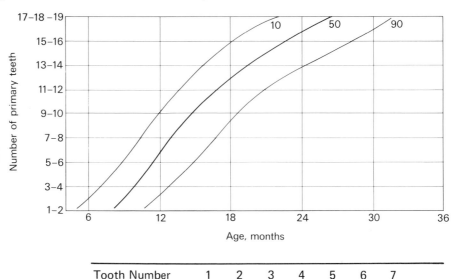

Figure 13.1 Centile chart for eruption of primary dentition. (Reproduced from Harvey and Parkinson (1977) *Journal of Maternal and Child Health*, **2**, 448, by permission of the authors and editors).

Figure 13.2 Approximate ages (in years to the nearest ½ year) of eruption of permanent teeth (Jackson and Fairpo 1976).

Tooth Number	1	2	3	4	5	6	7	
Maxillary	7	8	11	10	11	6	11½	Years
Mandibular	6	7	10	10½	11½	6	11½	Years

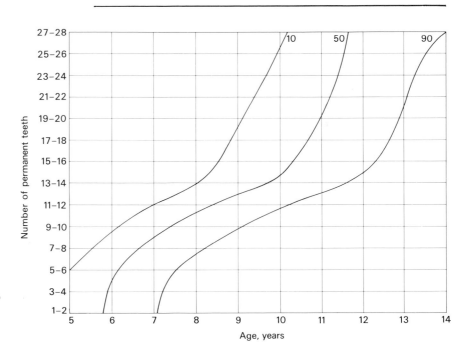

Figure 13.3 Centile chart for the eruption of permanent dentition (Jackson and Fairpo 1976).

14: Timetable of human embryonic development

Adverse influences which result in congenital malformations may be genetic or environmental. The former are active from conception, but at subsequent stages other teratogenic agents such as drugs, infections or maternal malnutrition may be implicated. These influences are more likely to have an effect at a time when the organ involved is developing actively embryologically, than when it is fully formed. It is therefore of value to know the stages of embryonic development, and these are listed in Figure 14.1 for the first two months of embryonic life (Smithells 1971). Fertilisation, which is the onset of embryonic development, occurs usually within 24 hours of ovulation, about 14 days after the beginning of the last menstrual period.

Days of embryonic life	Crown-rump length (mm)	General body form and skeletal system	Nervous system and sense organs	Cardiovascular and respiratory systems	Digestive system	Genito-urinary system
0	0	Ovum Zygote				
		Blastocyst Implantation				
10	1					
			Neural plate	Cardiogenic plate		
20	2	Somites		Heart tubes fuse 1st aortic arch	Fore and hindgut	
			Optic vesicles Otocyst		Liver bud	Pronephros Mesonephros
		Anterior limb buds Posterior limb buds	Anterior neuropore closes Posterior neuropore closes	Lung primordia Septum primum Aortic arches	Stomach primordium Dorsal pancreas	
30	4					
		Myotomes	Olfactory pits	Primary and lobar bronchi	Ventral pancreas Spleen	Metanephros Genital ridge
				Septum secundum I–V septum	Umbilical hernia Division of cloaca	
40	10					
		Finger rays Cartilaginous models	Primordium of cerebellum Retinal pigment Pinnae forming	Ductus venosus Division of truncus		Primordium of gonad
50	20	Primary ossification centres	Eyelids Semicircular canals	Septa complete Segmental bronchi	Rectum and bladder separated Lumen in gall bladder	Gonadal differentiation Müllerian primordium
		Separate digits Palatal processes grow medially	Differentiation of cerebral cortex			
				Main blood vessels present		Uterus complete Gonad differentiated
60	30				Umbilical hernia reduced	
		Palatal fusion				

Figure 14.1 Stages of embryonic development. (Reproduced from Smithells R. W. (1971) *Scientific Basis of Obstetrics and Gynaecology*, p. 252, ed. R. R. McDonald, published by Churchill Livingstone, Edinburgh, by permission of the author and editor.)

15: Gestational age assessment in the newborn

Birth weight may not be an accurate indication of gestational age, and it is important to distinguish different types of low birth weight babies. These include babies born preterm, i.e. less than 37 complete weeks gestation, whose weight may be appropriate for that length of gestation, and those whose weight is lighter than would be expected from their gestational age. Figures 12.1 and 12.3 show the centile distributions of weight (and length and head circumference) at various gestational ages (Gairdner and Pearson 1971). The measurements of a preterm baby are plotted at the appropriate number of weeks corresponding to gestational age. Later measurements are plotted at the appropriate intervals in relation to this initial record. Weights below the 10th centile are considered 'light for dates'.

Reasons for ascertaining gestational age of newborns

These include:

1 Evaluation of developmental progress later in infancy will clearly depend on the length of gestation at the time of birth.

2 Certain conditions are common in small babies that are preterm (e.g. feeding difficulties, hyperbilirubinaemia, respiratory problems, infections, brain-damage, haemorrhagic disease) and these differ from the problems particularly associated with babies that are light for dates (notably hypoglycaemia). Anticipation of these problems will affect management.

3 Babies whose gestational ages differ at birth may have different prospects for their future growth and development. Those that in addition to being light for dates have also a shorter length and smaller head circumference than expected are likely to have been subject to some adverse influence from an early age of gestation. Frequently the effect of this may persist postnatally as a retardation of growth or development or both.

Method of assessing gestational age of newborns

Assessment of gestational age based on the date of the mother's last menstrual period and other obstetric data is frequently unreliable. Clinical observations of newborn babies demonstrate many differences according to the length of gestation, and certain of these features have been selected to form the basis of simple methods of assessment.

Farr et al. (1966) described 11 external physical characteristics on the basis of which gestational age could be estimated to ±2.4 weeks with 95% confidence limits. Another group of criteria for assessment of length of gestation is based on neurological observations and though there is considerable variation in the ages at which neurological signs develop, incorporation of several of these criteria improves the accuracy of the assessment. Dubowitz et al. (1970) have described 10 neurological criteria which, in addition to the 11 external characteristics, improve the 95% confidence limits in evaluating gestational age to ±2.0 weeks. The details of these two sets of criteria and their scoring systems are shown in Figures 15.1 and 15.2. The total of these scores is used to estimate gestational age from the graph in Figure 15.3 (p. 82). This method should be undertaken within the first 48 hours of life and can be performed by an experienced observer in less than 10 minutes. Parkin et al. (1976) have pointed out that this method may prove difficult in ill babies when, in addition, neurological observations may be misleading. By selecting only 4 of the external criteria, they claim an accuracy of ± 15 days (with 95% confidence limits) in assessing gestational age at birth, even in ill babies. These 4 criteria are skin colour, skin texture, breast development and ear firmness, as included in Figure 15.1, and their graph (which is not a straight line) relating the total score to gestational age is shown in Figure 15.4 (p. 82). As one of these observations is skin colour, this method is not suitable for African or Asian babies. It is also unreliable for babies with gestational ages of less than 30 weeks, when examinations should be repeated at weekly intervals. A recent report (Woods and Malan 1977), in which gestational age assessment was undertaken on twins, has demonstrated a marked difference in these estimates based on external criteria (but not on neurological criteria) if there was a significant weight difference between the pair. External criteria alone may give a misleadingly low score for growth-retarded babies.

Facing page
Figure 15.1 External criteria for assessment of gestational age in the newborn infant (adapted from Farr *et al.* (1966), *Developmental Medicine and Child Neurology*, **8**, 507, by permission of the authors and editors).

EXTERNAL SIGN	SCORE 0	1	2	3	4
OEDEMA	Obvious oedema hands and feet; pitting over tibia	No obvious oedema hands and feet; pitting over tibia	No oedema		
SKIN TEXTURE	Very thin, gelatinous	Thin and smooth	Smooth; medium thickness. Rash or superficial peeling	Slight thickening. Superficial cracking and peeling esp. hands and feet	Thick and parchment-like; superficial or deep cracking
SKIN COLOUR (infant not crying)	Dark red	Uniformly pink	Pale pink: variable over body	Pale. Only pink over ears, lips, palms or soles	
SKIN OPACITY (trunk)	Numerous veins and venules clearly seen, especially over abdomen	Veins and tributaries seen	A few large vessels clearly seen over abdomen	A few large vessels seen indistinctly over abdomen	No blood vessels seen
LANUGO (over back)	No lanugo	Abundant; long and thick over whole back	Hair thinning especially over lower back	Small amount of lanugo and bald areas	At least half of back devoid of lanugo
PLANTAR CREASES	No skin creases	Faint red marks over anterior half of sole	Definite red marks over more than anterior half; indentations over less than anterior third	Indentations over more than anterior third	Definite deep indentations over more than anterior third
NIPPLE FORMATION	Nipple barely visible; no areola	Nipple well defined; areola smooth and flat diameter < 0.75 cm	Areola stippled, edge not raised; diameter < 0.75 cm	Areola stippled, edge raised diameter > 0.75 cm	
BREAST SIZE	No breast tissue palpable	Breast tissue on one or both sides < 0.5 cm diameter	Breast tissue both sides; one or both 0.5–1.0 cm diameter	Breast tissue both sides; one or both > 1 cm diameter	
EAR FORM	Pinna flat and shapeless, little or no incurving of edge	Incurving of part of edge of pinna	Partial incurving whole of upper pinna	Well-defined incurving whole of upper pinna	
EAR FIRMNESS	Pinna soft, easily folded, no recoil	Pinna soft, easily folded, slow recoil	Cartilage to edge of pinna, but soft in places, ready recoil	Pinna firm, cartilage to edge, instant recoil	
GENITALIA Male	Neither testis in scrotum	At least one testis high in scrotum	At least one testis right down		
Female (with hips half abducted)	Labia majora widely separated, labia minora protruding	Labia majora almost cover labia minora	Labia majora completely cover labia minora		

POSTURE. Observed with infant quiet and in supine position. Score 0: Arms and legs extended; 1: beginning of flexion of hips and knees, arms extended; 2: stronger flexion of legs, arms extended; 3: arms slightly flexed, legs flexed and abducted; 4: full flexion of arms and legs.

SQUARE WINDOW. The hand is flexed on the forearm between the thumb and index finger of the examiner. Enough pressure is applied to get as full a flexion as possible, and the angle between the hypothenar eminence and the ventral aspect of the forearm is measured and graded according to diagram. (Care is taken not to rotate the infant's wrist while doing this manoeuvre.)

ANKLE DORSIFLEXION. The foot is dorsiflexed onto the anterior aspect of the leg, with the examiner's thumb on the sole of the foot and other fingers behind the leg. Enough pressure is applied to get as full flexion as possible, and the angle between the dorsum of the foot and the anterior aspect of the leg is measured.

ARM RECOIL. With the infant in the supine position the forearms are first flexed for 5 seconds, then fully extended by pulling on the hands, and then released. The sign is fully positive if the arms return briskly to full flexion (Score 2). If the arms return to incomplete flexion or the response is sluggish it is graded as Score 1. If they remain extended or are only followed by random movements the score is 0.

LEG RECOIL. With the infant supine, the hips and knees are fully flexed for 5 seconds, then extended by traction on the feet, and released. A maximal response is one of full flexion of the hips and knees (Score 2). A partial flexion scores 1, and minimal or no movement scores 0.

POPLITEAL ANGLE. With the infant supine and his pelvis flat on the examining couch, the thigh is held in the knee-chest position by the examiner's left index finger and thumb supporting the knee. The leg is then extended by gentle pressure from the examiner's right index finger behind the ankle and the popliteal angle is measured.

HEEL TO EAR MANOEUVRE. With the baby supine, draw the baby's foot as near to the head as it will go without forcing it. Observe the distance between the foot and the head as well as the degree of extension at the knee. Grade according to diagram. Note that the knee is left free and may draw down alongside the abdomen.

SCARF SIGN. With the baby supine, take the infant's hand and try to put it around the neck and as far posteriorly as possible around the opposite shoulder. Assist this manoeuvre by lifting the elbow across the body. See how far the elbow will go across and grade according to illustrations. Score 0: Elbow reaches opposite axillary line; 1: Elbow between midline and opposite axillary line; 2: Elbow reaches midline; 3: Elbow will not reach midline.

HEAD LAG. With the baby lying supine, grasp the hands (or the arms if a very small infant) and pull him slowly towards the sitting position. Observe the position of the head in relation to the trunk and grade accordingly. In a small infant the head may initially be supported by one hand. Score 0: Complete lag; 1: Partial head control; 2: Able to maintain head in line with body; 3: Brings head anterior to body.

VENTRAL SUSPENSION. The infant is suspended in the prone position, with examiner's hand under the infant's chest (one hand in a small infant, two in a large infant). Observe the degree of extension of the back and the amount of flexion of the arms and legs. Also note the relation of the head to the trunk. Grade according to diagrams.

If the score for an individual criterion differs on the two sides of the baby, take the mean.

Figure 15.2 (above and facing) Neurological criteria for assessment of gestational age in the newborn infant (from Dubowitz, Lilly M. S., Dubowitz, Victor and Goldberg, Cissie (1970) Clinical assessment of gestational age in the newborn infant, *Journal of Paediatrics*, **77**, 4–5, by permission of authors and editors).

Neurological sign	Score					
	0	1	2	3	4	5
Posture						
Square window	90°	60°	45°	30°	0°	
Ankle dorsiflexion	90°	75°	45°	20°	0°	
Arm recoil	180°	90–180°	< 90°			
Leg recoil	180°	90–180°	< 90°			
Popliteal angle	180°	160°	130°	110°	90°	< 90°
Heel to ear						
Scarf sign						
Head lag						
Ventral suspension						

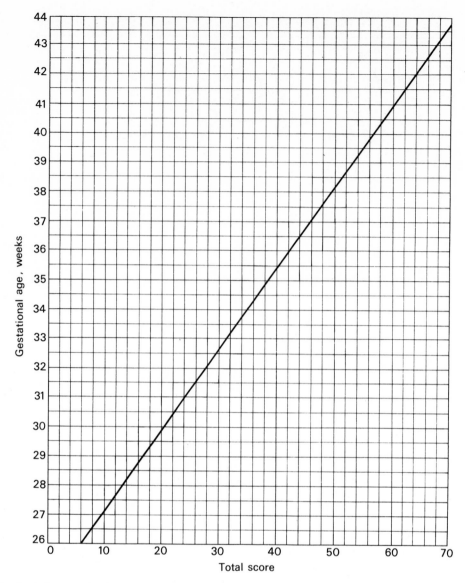

Figure 15.3 Graph relating gestational age to total score of criteria (from Dubowitz, Lilly M. S., Dubowitz, Victor and Goldberg, Cissie (1970) Clinical assessment of gestational age in the newborn infant. *Journal of Paediatrics*, **77**, 10, by permission of authors and editors).

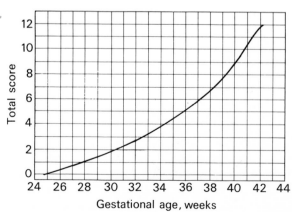

Figure 15.4 Graph relating gestational age to total score for 4 selected external criteria (from Parkin *et al.* (1976) *Archives of Disease in Childhood*, **51**, 259, by permission of the authors and editors).

16: Developmental assessment

A knowledge of the normal pattern of development in infants and young children is an essential requirement for every paediatrician, though in older children fuller evaluation of intelligence requires the experience of an educational psychologist. It is important at any age to be able to recognise those children whose progress and performance are sufficiently outside the normal range to indicate the need for more precise evaluation. The earlier defects are recognised, whether physical, developmental or psychological, the better the outlook with correct management and appropriate placement. Nevertheless, it is important not to diagnose developmental delay when it is not really there, and so attach a diagnostic label with all the consequent implications. Certain children will be at greater risk of defects and warrant careful observation, such as those with preceding disease, ante-, peri- or post-natal, those with congenital anomalies, neurological abnormalities, relevant family histories, behaviour disorders, etc.

Development of the Infant and Young Child

Assessment is based both on observations of the child's performance at the time, including a full examination, and on information about the previous pattern and rate of development as indicated by a history from someone else, usually the parents.

In evaluating a young child's development, as in assessing intelligence in older children, many factors which may influence performance must be taken into consideration. These include the nature of the environment, the child's physical wellbeing, and his co-operation at the time of examination. Ideally the infant or young child should be in good health, not hungry, fatigued or on sedative drugs, not distracted by background noise or movement and not distressed by separation (so preferably accompanied by mother). Observations only show how a child behaved on one particular day, when circumstances may not have been optimal, and ideally repeat observations are required. Only as a result of long term assessment can a reliable prediction of future performance and ultimate mental ability be given. Observations over a short period of time merely indicate what point a child's development has reached then in comparison with the average child of the same age. This, together with appropriate provision of treatment, is the essential purpose of a developmental assessment, and not to foretell future intelligence. Gross deviations from the normal are likely to be of significance and probably of predictive value, but the more precise ultimate outcome will be dependent on many other factors, notably environmental circumstances and the general state of health and wellbeing.

Several writers have studied the development of normal children, and the abridged report of Sheridan (1968) is particularly useful and convenient. This details the performance of normal children at various ages in four different fields: posture and gross movement, vision and fine movement, hearing and speech, social behaviour and play. Based on this system, selected, easily evaluated examples showing the average ages of acquiring various abilities are listed in Figure 16.1. Such a list is only a guideline for, as with physical growth, the variations in developmental progress in normal children are considerable. It is important with young children to take into consideration the length of gestation at the time of birth. Stages of development are stepping stones which lead one to another rather than milestones, so that one ability cannot be acquired until the previous one is mastered. Thus the sequence of events in most children is usually the same, though the rate of progress may vary from child to child. However, occasionally a step may be missed out and progress may be erratic with slow and rapid phases. Mental retardation is usually indicated by a deficit in all these four categories of development, and a defect in only one may indicate a motor or sensory abnormality in an isolated field, but may merely be a variant of normal. The particular field in which the defect is suspected will then require fuller investigation.

There is a considerable range in the ages at which normal children are first able to perform various activities and the extent of this range is much greater with some functions than with others. This was shown by the 'Denver Developmental Screening Test' (see Appendix, p. 100), based on observations on over 1000 normal children in Denver aged 2 weeks to 6 years (Frankenburg and Dodds 1967). 105 test items were selected, classified into the same four groups as those of Sheridan. This test has formed a useful screening procedure indicating whether a child's performance falls within the normal range. Differences were found in the ages at which boys and girls were able to perform particular test items, and also differences between children of parents of different occupational groups. Strictly these observations only reflect the population of Denver, and subsequent studies such as the Cardiff report (Bryant *et*

AGE	POSTURE AND GROSS MOVEMENT		VISION AND FINE MOVEMENT				HEARING AND SPEECH		SOCIAL BEHAVIOUR AND PLAY
			VISION	FINE MOVEMENT	CUBES (1 inch)	DRAWING/COPYING	HEARING	SPEECH	
6 WEEKS	PRONE HEAD CONTROL	Chin raised momentarily. Pelvis flat. Head held momentarily in same plane as body.	Turns head and eyes to light. Fixates on objects and follows them.				Startles to sound.		Smiles (in response to mother).
3 MONTHS	PRONE HEAD CONTROL HELD SITTING HELD STANDING	Head and chest lifted up—supported with forearms. Almost complete, only slight head lag. Back straight, head mostly held up but tends to bob forward. Sags at the knees.	Follows toy at 6–10 in. Hand regard.	Hands loosely open.			Quietens to pleasing sounds. Turns eyes towards sound.	Vocalises when pleased. Chuckles and coos.	Laughs (3–4 months)
6 MONTHS	SUPINE PRONE SITS HELD STANDING	Raises head. Supports on extended arms. Rolls from front to back. with support and momentarily alone. Bears weight on feet. Bounces up and down.	Moves head and eyes in all directions. Squint abnormal (after 4 months) Watches rolling balls at 10 ft	Uses whole hand in palmar grasp (ulnar approach). Transfers.			Turns to soft sounds 18 in. from either ear.	Single or double syllables.	Still friendly with strangers. Reaches for toys. Does not look for lost toy. Takes everything to mouth.
9 MONTHS	SITS CRAWL STANDS	unsupported for 10 minutes. attempts with support momentarily and steps purposefully. Pulls to stand.	Looks for dropped toys.	Scissor grasp between index and thumb.			Localises soft sounds at 3 ft, and above and below ear level. Understands 'no' and 'bye-bye'.	Babbles tunefully. Vocalises deliberately to attract attention.	Cries if handled by strangers. Pat-a-cake. Waves bye-bye. Peek-a-boo. Chews solids.
1 YEAR	SITS CRAWLS WALKS STANDS	well, indefinitely on all fours. round furniture and holding one or both hands. alone momentarily.	Points with index finger at objects of interest.	Precise pincer grasp between index and thumb. Index approach.			Localises sound above head. Understands simple commands. Knows name.	2–3 words with meaning.	Shy. Co-operates with dressing (arms out). Gives toys to mother. Drops toys deliberately.
15 MONTHS	CRAWLS WALKS	upstairs unaided on wide base (10 steps from 13 months). Can get to standing position unaided.			Builds tower of 2 cubes.			Continual jabber and jargon. 2–6 recognisable words	Holds cup and drinks from it. No longer mouthing.

Age	Posture and large movements	Vision and fine movements	Hearing and speech	Social behaviour
18 MONTHS	WALKS alone pulling or pushing toy. Walks upstairs one hand held or holding rail.	Scribbles. Hand preference beginning.	Jargon. 6–20 recognisable words.	Co-operates with feeding and uses spoon. Emotionally dependent on familiar adult. Takes off socks, shoes, gloves. Throws ball. Bowel control.
2 YEARS	WALKS up and downstairs holding on—2 feet to a step. Picks up toy without falling. RUNS safely on whole foot.	Turns pages singly. Definite hand preference. Builds tower of 6 cubes. Copies | or —	50 or more words. Joins 2–3 words to convey ideas.	Plays near other children but not with them. Clings to mother. Puts on and takes off shoes and socks. Dry by day.
2½ YEARS	WALKS upstairs alone. Walks on tiptoe. JUMPS with both feet. Kicks large ball.	Tower of 8 cubes. Forms train.	Over 200 words. Knows full name, I, me and you.	Still dependent emotionally on adults. Recognises self in pictures.
3 YEARS	WALKS upstairs 1 foot per step, downstairs 2 feet per step. STANDS on one foot momentarily. Rides tricycle.	Tower of 9 cubes. Copies bridge. Copies O. Beginning to draw man with head.	Asks questions. Simple conversations. Says 'I' not 'me'. Nursery rhymes. Seldom stutters.	Feeds with spoon and fork. Joins in play with others. Dresses fully (except buttons). Affectionate. Dry by night.
4 YEARS	WALKS up and downstairs 1 foot per step. STANDS on 1 foot a few seconds.	Buttons clothes. Builds 3 steps from 6 cubes after demonstration. Copies +. Draws man with head, legs and trunk.	Conversation fluent. Home address. Usually has stopped lisping.	Needs other children to play. Self-willed. Dresses and undresses with help.
5 YEARS	SKIPS on alternate feet. RUNS on toes.	Builds 3 steps from 6 cubes (from model). Copies □ (4½). Copies △ (5). Copies ◇ (6). Draws recognisable man and house (4½).	Gives age. Few infantile substitutions.	Uses knife and fork. Dresses and undresses alone. Washes and dries face and hands.

Figure 16.1 Stages of development in the average infant and young child.

al. 1974) do show minor differences dependent on the population selected. Nevertheless the Denver Test has proved a useful simple guideline applicable to young children in this age range.

Normal Reflexes and Responses in Early Childhood

The normally developing child demonstrates various reflexes and reactions which appear and disappear in a recognised sequence. The most consistent of these reflexes are described in Figure 16.3. This also shows the usual ages at which they may be expected to appear and disappear. These reflexes may be separated into groups. Primitive reflexes are present at birth or in early months, but gradually become more difficult to elicit, or weaker, and ultimately disappear as cortical control develops. The loss of certain of these reflexes is necessary for the development of other reflexes which appear later and are retained through life, and form the basis of normal posture and more highly differentiated movement patterns. Certain 'permanent' reflexes are present from birth and throughout life.

When reflexes and reactions are being observed and interpreted, the baby should be awake, but quiet and not crying. Because asymmetry of reflexes is very significant, the baby should be positioned symmetrically with the head in the midline. Abnormalities of reflex patterns may be shown by their being exaggerated, diminished, asymmetrical or delayed in age of onset or disappearance. Such findings suggest cerebral damage or abnormalities of brain development.

Intelligence Assessment of Older Children

It is beyond the scope of this book to consider in detail methods of evaluating intelligence. Paediatricians, on the basis of their observations and the history of development, will be able to recognise those children who need fuller assessment and will refer appropriately. It should be recognised, however, that testing requires co-operation of the child, and a satisfactory performance requires the child to have adequate experience, attention span, and the ability to see, hear and communicate or perform as requested. (It is impossible to assess intelligence satisfactorily in a handicapped child without recognising that the handicap itself is bound to affect performance.)

Draw-a-Man Test

This test provides one method of measuring levels of mental development of children between the ages of 3 and 10 years. It is easy to undertake and score and, though approximate, shows a significant degree of correlation with other tests of mental age.

The child is asked to draw a man as carefully and completely as possible. He is allowed as much time as he wants and is left alone and undisturbed.

The modified simpler test uses only 28 criteria for scoring, listed in Figure 16.2 (1 to 28) Bakwin *et al.* 1948). This is sufficient for testing the pre-school child; the fuller original test of Goodenough (1926) comprises 51 criteria, the extra 23 (29 to 51) demonstrating proportion, facial detail and motor coordination of the child and is suitable for an older child (see also Silver, 1950).

Scoring

In determining the mental age of a child, the basal age is 3 years. For each criterion met by the drawing the child is credited with an additional 3 months, and the total so credited is added to the basal age to give the mental age.

Interpretation

The test requires the child to visualise the human figure, to organise and interpret his concept and reproduce it by motor skills. It thus serves not only as a basic guideline for measuring mental age, but as a diagnostic aid, as it may indicate defects of vision, of neuromuscular control or of interpretation, possibly caused by emotional upset (Coleman *et al.* 1959). Caution should be exercised in evaluating very poor drawings which could indicate such defects rather than necessarily low intelligence. High scores may occur in children with schizophrenia. Ability is clearly influenced by experience and practice.

1 Head present.
2 Legs present.
3 Arms present.
4 Trunk present.
5 Length of trunk greater than breadth.
6 Shoulder indicated.
7 Both arms and legs attached to trunk.
8 Legs attached to trunk and arms to trunk at correct point.
9 Neck present.
10 Outline of neck continuous with that of head or trunk or both.
11 Eyes present.
12 Nose present.
13 Mouth present.
14 Both nose and mouth in two dimensions; two lips shown.
15 Nostrils indicated.
16 Hair shown.
17 Hair on more than circumference of head, non-transparent, better than scribble.
18 Clothing present.
19 Two articles of clothing, non-transparent.
20 Entire drawing, with sleeves and trousers shown, free from transparency.
21 Four or more articles of clothing definitely indicated.
22 Costume complete without incongruities.
23 Fingers shown.
24 Correct number of fingers shown.
25 Fingers in two dimensions, length greater than breadth, angle subtended not greater than 180 degrees.
26 Opposition of thumbs shown.
27 Hand shown as distinct from fingers or arms.
28 Arm joint shown, elbow, shoulder or both.

29 Leg joint shown, knee, hip or both.
30 Head in proportion.
31 Arms in proportion.
32 Legs in proportion.
33 Feet in proportion.
34 Both arms and legs in two dimensions.
35 Heel shown.
36 Firm lines without overlapping.
37 Firm lines with correct joining.
38 Head outline more than a circle.
39 Trunk outline more than a circle.
40 Outline of arms and legs without narrowing at junction of body.
41 Features symmetrical and in correct position.
42 Ears present.
43 Ears in correct position and proportion.
44 Eyebrows or lashes.
45 Pupils of eye.
46 Eye length greater than height.
47 Eye glance directed to front in profile.
48 Both chin and forehead shown.
49 Projection of chin shown.
50 Profile with not more than one error.
51 Correct profile.

Figure 16.2 Draw-a-man Test — criteria for scoring.

REFLEX	DESCRIPTION	COMMENTS
	PRIMITIVE REFLEXES	
Moro Response	Baby lies supine with the head supported in one hand a little off the table and then released suddenly. This causes abduction and extension of the arms with opening of the hands, often followed by adduction of the arms and crying.	Pathology may cause delay in onset or disappearance, exaggerated, decreased or asymmetrical responses. The reflex is present at birth even in preterm babies —complete from 37 weeks gestation but weaker and less complete before.
Galant's Reflex (trunk incurvation)	Baby held in ventral suspension, stimulation of the skin down the back lateral to the spine results in flexion of the spine to the stimulated side.	This reflex is present in very preterm babies.
Placing Reflex	When the dorsal aspect of the foot is brought against a table edge, the leg is raised to step on the table.	The reflex present at birth is slightly delayed in small preterm babies. From about 5–9 months the response becomes less brisk in about 50% of babies, but subsequently is accompanied by weight bearing.
Stepping Reflex	Baby held vertical over a table with the soles of feet pressed against it, causes stepping movements of the legs.	This reflex must be lost before voluntary walking can occur. Present at birth, it is delayed in small preterm babies.
Palmar Grasp	Insertion of an object into the palm from the ulnar side results in flexion of the fingers and grasping of object.	The reflex is present at birth but delayed in preterm babies. It becomes progressively weaker, prior to loss after 3 months, before the hand can be used for support.
Plantar Grasp	Stroking the sole behind the toes causes flexion of the toes.	The reflex is lost when the foot can bear weight. It becomes progressively weaker from 9 months and is seldom elicitable after 12 months.
Crossed Extension Reflex	One leg is held fully extended and on stroking the sole of that foot, the opposite leg flexes, adducts and then extends.	The reflex is present at birth, even in preterm babies, though incomplete in those of less than 37 weeks gestation. It gradually merges into an active defence pattern.
Asymmetrical Tonic Neck Reflex	Baby lying supine, when the head faces or is turned to one side, the arm and leg on that side extend and on the opposite side flex.	Usually incomplete and weak in normal babies but most obvious at about 3 months. The reflex may prevent rolling over in early weeks and must be lost in order to do so, or for the hands to be brought to the face. Becomes progressively weaker prior to disappearance.
Symmetrical Tonic Neck Reflex	On all fours, extension of the neck causes extension of the arms and flexion of the legs; flexion of the neck causes the reverse.	The reflex appears for a short period about 6 months, just before starting to crawl, but must be lost in order to crawl effectively.
Landau Reflex	Held in ventral suspension, the head, spine and legs extend. Depression of head causes flexion of hips, knees and elbows.	The reflex becomes difficult to elicit after 12 months. There is great variability in the pattern of this response.

Figure 16.3 Normal reflexes in early childhood and average ages of appearance and disappearance.

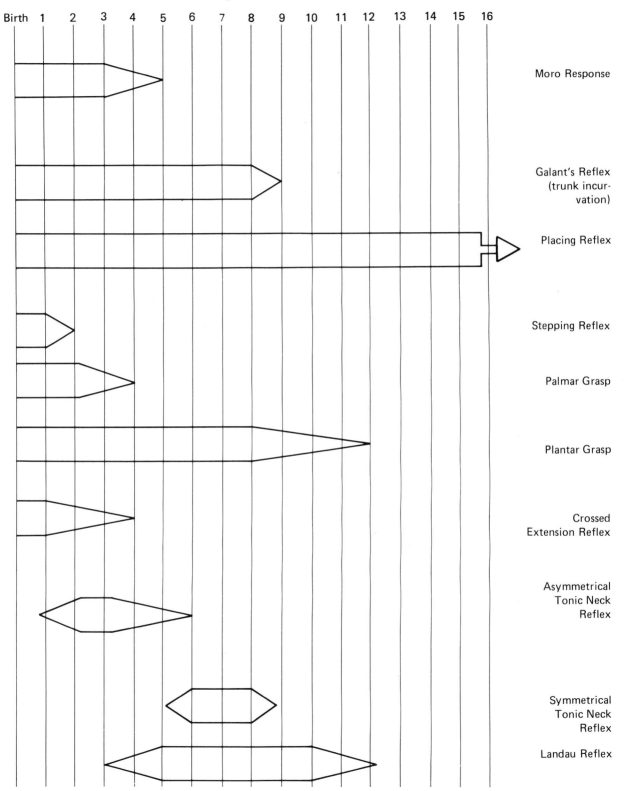

Age in months

| | Birth | 1 | 2 | 3 | 4 | 5 | 6 | 7 | 8 | 9 | 10 | 11 | 12 | 13 | 14 | 15 | 16 |

Moro Response

Galant's Reflex (trunk incurvation)

Placing Reflex

Stepping Reflex

Palmar Grasp

Plantar Grasp

Crossed Extension Reflex

Asymmetrical Tonic Neck Reflex

Symmetrical Tonic Neck Reflex

Landau Reflex

REFLEX	DESCRIPTION	COMMENTS

REFLEXES WHICH DEVELOP POSTNATALLY AND PERSIST

REFLEX	DESCRIPTION	COMMENTS
Leg Straightening Reflex	When the sole of the foot is pressed on the table, the legs and body straighten.	The reflex is lost at about 2 months but re-appears when plantar grasp disappears, at 6–8 months.
Balance Reaction —Sitting	Tilting a child in the sitting position side-ways or backwards causes extension of the arm to prevent falling.	This reflex appears about 6 months and is necessary for stable sitting.
Balance Reaction —Standing	Pushing the standing child laterally causes extension of arm and leg to prevent falling.	This reflex appears about 6 months and is necessary for standing.
Parachute Reaction	The child held in ventral suspension is sud-denly lowered head first towards a table. The arms extend as protection.	The reflex appears about 6 months and persists through life. The name is derived from the French word 'chute'.

PERMANENT REFLEXES

REFLEX	DESCRIPTION	COMMENTS
Plantar Reflex (Babinski)	Scratching of the lateral aspect of the plan-tar surface of the foot from the heel for-wards causes flexion of the great toe. In infancy the normal response is usually extensor associated with fanning of the other toes, but after 2 years such a response is pathological.	Pathology may be shown by asymmetry. The reflex is extensor from birth, usually becoming flexor between 12 and 18 months.
Tendon Jerks	In babies the knee and biceps jerks are the most easily elicited.	Exaggerated responses may be elicited by tapping progressively further from the site of the tendon.

Figure 16.3 Normal reflexes in early childhood and average ages of appearance and disappearance.

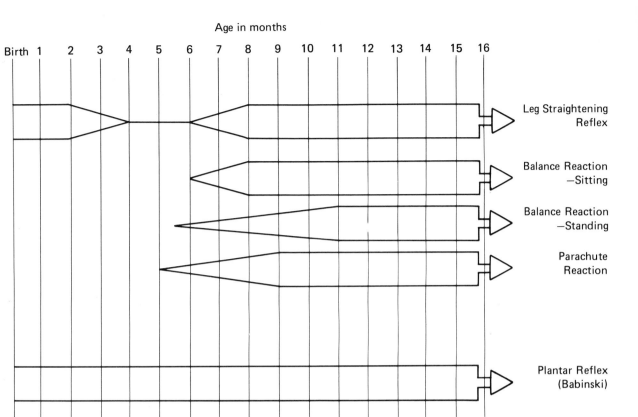

Age in months

| Birth | 1 | 2 | 3 | 4 | 5 | 6 | 7 | 8 | 9 | 10 | 11 | 12 | 13 | 14 | 15 | 16 |

Leg Straightening Reflex

Balance Reaction —Sitting

Balance Reaction —Standing

Parachute Reaction

Plantar Reflex (Babinski)

Tendon Jerks

17: Ventilatory function

Peak expiratory flow rate

Comprehensive testing of pulmonary function in children is not practical as a routine investigation for most paediatricians. Much information can be obtained, however, from a single lung function — peak expiratory flow rate (PEFR) — which is reduced in conditions of lower airway obstruction, as in many childhood pulmonary disorders, and is very simple to estimate in outpatients or on the ward.

Technique

Peak expiratory flow rate is estimated by means of a Wright Peak Flow Meter. The technique is explained fully to the child who, when sitting upright comfortably, holds the apparatus with the mouthpiece horizontal and the dial vertical and facing the right. He then inspires deeply and, applying his lips firmly around the mouthpiece, blows out with as short and sharp an expiration as possible. Unless the child is accustomed to the procedure, several attempts may be required (with adequate rest between) to achieve an acceptable result, depending on the understanding and ability to co-operate. Usually the average of two highest satisfactory readings is accepted.

It is usually possible to obtain valid results with children over 5 years, and sometimes younger, but a smaller instrument is normally required for children under 6 or those who are particularly disabled. This small model is calibrated over a range 20–200 litres per minute in contrast to the standard apparatus with a range of 60–1000 litres per minute.

A graph obtained from tests on normal boys and girls (Godfrey *et al.* 1970) is shown in Figure 17.1 and provides a normal range of values (± 2 S.D.) appropriate for height. The figure also shows normal values for forced vital capacity (FVC) and forced expiratory volume in 1 second (FEV$_1$). Analysis of results of several series has shown that simple respiratory function tests correlate as well with height as with any other physical variable.

Application

Peak flow estimations are of value in the following circumstances:

1 In diseases of the lower airway, where knowledge of the degree of obstruction is of value in diagnosis and management. The commonest application in childhood is in asthma. Serial observations indicate progress of the disease in an acute episode or at intervals in longer term follow up. It is useful in assessing the efficacy of various forms of treatment, both as an immediate response or long term.

2 As an aid in evaluating the degree of ventilatory impairment in neuro-muscular (and occasionally skeletal) disorders which may impair chest expansion.

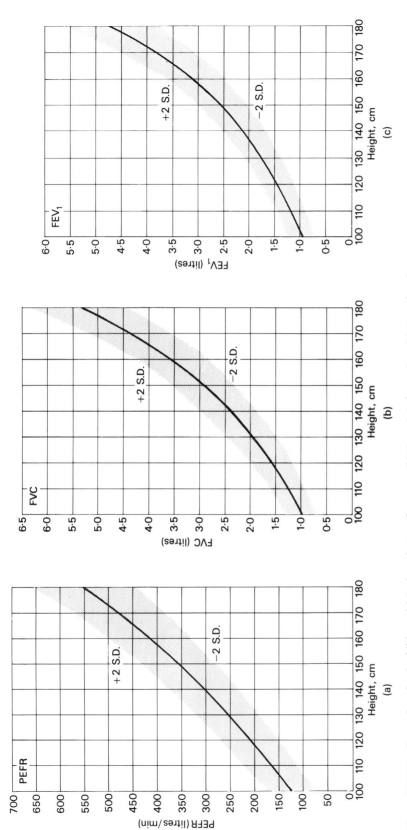

Figure 17.1 Ventilatory function in children. (a) Peak expiratory flow rate. (b) Forced vital capacity. (c) Forced expiratory volume in 1 second. (Based on the data of Godfrey et al. (1970) *British Journal of Diseases of the Chest*, **64**, 15, by permission of the authors and publishers.)

18: Electrocardiography, pulse rate and blood pressure

Electrocardiography

Interpretation of electrocardiograms in children presents difficulties because of the variation in the pattern with age, with size of the child, with the shape and thickness of the chest wall and in some respects (such as QT interval) with heart rate. For satisfactory records the infant or child should be quiet, and in infants this may be achieved while feeding or sucking or by the mother holding the child in her lap.

Electrode placing

Deflections may be distorted as the result of excessive electrode jelly on the skin of infants and children. Because of its thinness the skin has lower resistance than that of adults and very little jelly is required. Electrodes for chest leads in children should be 1.5 cm in diameter as larger adult size electrodes cause further conduction defects. Limb electrodes may be more conveniently placed on upper arms or thighs rather than wrists or ankles.

   Precordial lead positions are as follows:

V_1 — 4th intercostal space — right sternal border
V_2 — 4th intercostal space — left sternal border
V_3 — midway between V_2 and V_4
V_4 — left 5th intercostal space — mid-clavicular line
V_5 — level of V_4 — anterior axillary line
V_6 — level of V_4 and V_5 — mid-axillary line
V_3R — as V_3 but to the right of the sternum
V_4R — as V_4 but to the right of the sternum.

Measurement

Measurement from the electrocardiogram is illustrated in Figure 18.1 (Jordan and Scott 1973). The paper is marked at 1 mm and 5 mm intervals. The paper speed should be 25 mm per second, and the machine standardised so that a potential of 1 mV produces a deflection of 10 mm. This can be halved with large deflections so that 1 mV produces a deflection of 5 mm.

Interpretation

Interpretation depends on the acceptance of a wide range of normality varying with factors indicated

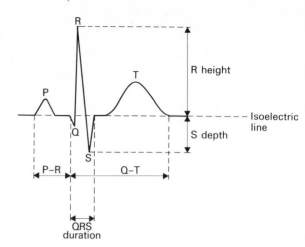

Figure 18.1 Measurement from the electrocardiogram. Note that the P-R interval is measured from the start of the P wave to the start of the QRS complex; the Q-T interval from the start of the QRS to the end of the T. (From Jordan and Scott (1973) *Heart Disease in Paediatrics*, p. 32, published by Butterworths, reproduced by permission of the authors and publisher.)

above, but average values for the duration, magnitude and pattern of the various components of the electrocardiogram and their alterations with age are shown in Figure 18.2, (based on data from Ziegler 1951). The values in brackets indicate normal ranges (approximately 3rd–97th centile range). These values would obviously require interpretation in the light of other clinical and radiological observations.

   The electrical axis of the heart is the direction in which electrical activity spreads through the ventricles. In the frontal plane this is indicated by the pattern of the QRS complexes in the limb leads, and can be estimated approximately from this pattern in leads 1 and 2 or leads 1 and AVf — as explained in Figure 18.3 (Jordan and Scott 1973). The horizontal plane can similarly be calculated from the chest leads, the transition zone between right and left ventricles being the lead where there are equal R and S waves.

Pulse rate and blood pressure

Through the years of childhood resting pulse rate steadily falls and blood pressure slightly rises up to the age of adolescence. Figure 18.4 indicates expected values and is a composite table compiled from many sources. There is little difference in the values for boys and girls.

	DURATION (seconds) Infancy → Adolescence		MAGNITUDE OR RANGE				PATTERN
			Birth	6 months	1 year	10 year / Adolescence	
P WAVE	0.05 (0.04–0.07) gradually increasing to 0.08 (0.06–0.10)		←————— 2.5 mm upper limit of normal —————→				Tallest P waves in leads 2, V_4R and V_1.
PR INTERVAL	0.10 (0.07–0.13) gradually increasing to 0.14 (0.10–0.19)						
QRS WAVE	0.07 (0.06–0.08)						
Q WAVE mm			←— 2–3 mm ——— 4 mm upper limit of normal —→				Present in leads 2, 3, AVF, V_5 and V_6. Abnormal in other leads.
R WAVE mm		V_4R V_1 V_5 V_6	8(4–12) 15(5–25) 12(2–25) 5(1–13)	5(2–7) 11(3–18) 20(10–28) 12(5–20)	4(0–7) 9(2–16) 20(10–30) 12(4–20)	2.5(0–6) / — ; 6(1–15) / 5(0–15) ; 20(10–40) / 18(8–30) ; 14(10–20) / 14(8–20)	Right Axis Deviation: Lead 1: Small R wave, large S wave. Lead 2 & 3: Large R wave, small S wave.
S WAVE mm		V_1 V_6	10(0–20) 6(0–15)	8(3–15) 2(0–5)	10(1–25) 1(0–4)	14(5–25) / 15(5–25) ; 1(0–5) / 1(0–5)	Left Axis Deviation: Lead 1: Large R, Small S, Frequently Q. Lead 3: Small R wave, large S wave.
QRS AXIS (Frontal Plane)			+135° (+90° to +180°)	+65° (+45° to +105°)	+60° (+20° to +100°)	+65° (+30° to +100°) / +65° (+30° to +100°)	Transition zone between R & L ventricles is at V_3 — S larger than R in V_4 = clockwise rotation. R larger than S in V_2 = anticlockwise rot'n.
HORIZONTAL PLANE AXIS							
QT INTERVAL	0.25 (0.2–0.3) gradually increasing to 0.35 (0.3–0.4)						
T WAVE	0.12 gradually increasing to 0.16 mean 0.14 (0.1–0.2)		1/4 to 1/3 of magnitude of R waves in leads with predominant R				After Day 3 inverted in AVR, V_4R, V_1 and usually V_2 and V_3 in early childhood. Becomes upright in V_2 and V_3 between 5 and 15 years. Inverted in AVL in vertical heart and lead 3 in horizontal. Inverted T in other leads abnormal.

Figure 18.2 Average values for components of electrocardiograms of children (based on data from Ziegler (1951) *Electrocardiographic Studies in Normal Infants and Children*, courtesy of Charles C. Thomas, Publisher, Springfield, Illinois).

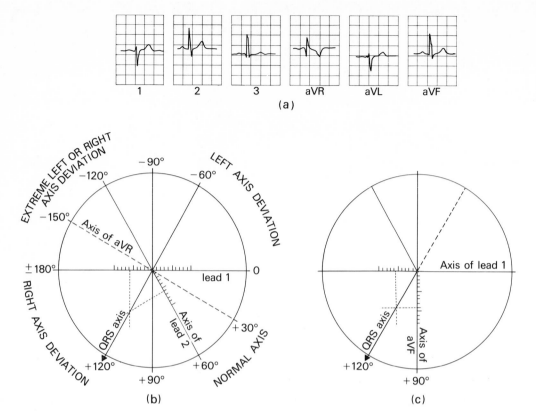

Figure 18.3 Calculation of the QRS axis (in the frontal plane). (a) Recordings or readings in various leads. (b) Using leads 1 and 2. Measure the height of R in lead 1 (2 mm) and subtract the depth of S (8 mm). Plot the answer (−6) along the axis of lead 1, which is horizontal (0°) in arbitrary units. In lead 2, R − S = 9 − 3 = + 6 which is plotted on the axis of lead 2, which is at 60°. Drop perpendiculars from these axes and the line from the origin through the intersection is the electrical axis. (c) The same calculation, using aVF instead of lead 2. This has the advantage that it is at right angles to lead 1, but the result of R − S (10 − 3 = 7) has to be multiplied by a factor, 1·3, to allow for the fact that aVF is an augmented unipolar lead and not, like lead 1, a bipolar lead. (A rough method is to look for a lead where R and S are nearly equal, in this case aVR. The axis will be at right angles to the axis of that lead, and it will be clear from examining one other lead in which direction it points.) (From Jordan and Scott (1973) *Heart Disease in Paediatrics*, p. 35, published by Butterworth & Co and reproduced by permission of the authors and publishers.)

Age	Resting Heart Rate (per minute)	Arterial Blood Pressure* mm Hg.	
		Systolic	Diastolic
1 day–1 month	110–150	70–80	
1 month	110–150	80	45
6–12 months	110–140	90	60
1 year	100–140	95	60
2 years	85–125	95	60
6 years	70–110	95	60
8 years	85–100	100	65
10 years	85–100	105	65
14 years	75– 90	115	65

Figure 18.4 Heart rate and arterial blood pressure values in normal children. (*Approximate mean values. S.D. is about 10 mm Hg at all ages.)

19: Kidney size and urine volume

Kidney size

Kidney outline can be demonstrated radiologically in 70–80% of children by plain abdominal X-ray. A supine film with focussing on the renal areas without special preparation is usually adequate. In the minority where this is not satisfactory, tomography or intravenous pyelography may be required.

Statistically it has been shown that kidney size correlates as well with body length or height during infancy and childhood as with other more complicated variables. Before puberty kidney size is well related to age, but in view of the marked variation in the age, magnitude and duration of the pubertal growth spurt, age is not overall as satisfactory as height for standardising kidney size. There is considerable variation in the size of normal kidneys, and in addition normal left and right kidneys may differ in length by as much as 5 mm. Figure 19.1 plots kidney length against body height, showing the mean

values for the population and the range of ± 1 S.D. (68% population) and ± 2½ S.D. (99% population). These values were based on intravenous pyelogram studies on children whose kidneys were considered to be normal (Hodson *et al.* 1962). Kidney length is the maximum length of the kidney and is a good indication of overall kidney size.

Despite the great range of kidney length within a normal population, knowledge of the size of kidneys and serial measurements to indicate rate of growth are of considerable value in diagnosing kidney disorders, in monitoring progress of disease, and indicating the extent to which both kidneys may be involved.

Urine volume

Figure 19.2 indicates urine volumes produced in 24-hour periods by normal children. The data are derived from several sources.

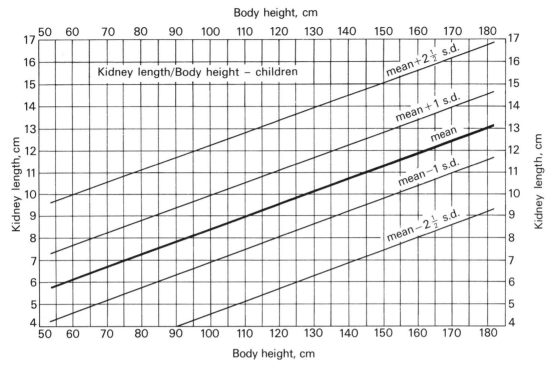

Figure 19.1 Graph relating kidney length and body height in childhood (reproduced with permission of Kodak Ltd, based on the data of Hodson *et al.* (1962) *Archives of Disease in Childhood*, 37, 616).

Age	Volume* (ml per 24 hours)
1–2 days	15–60
3–10 days	100–300
10 days–2 months	250–450
2 months–1 year	400–500
1 year–3 years	500–600
3 years–5 years	600–750
5 years–8 years	650–1000
>8 years	700–1500

Figure 19.2 24-hour urine volumes in normal children (*this range covers 95% of observed values).

Appendix: Equipment and suppliers

1. Growth Charts

The following charts are obtainable from:
Castlemead Publications,
(Publishing Division of Creaseys of Hertford Ltd),
Castlemead, Gascoyne Way, Hertford SG14 1LH

Growth records

Height and Weight	Boys	Girls
Attained		
0–5 years	SHWB 28	SHWG 29
0–19 years	GDB 11A	GDG 12A
Standards for Height		
Parents allowed for		
2–9 years	SCHB 16	SCHG 15
Height and Weight		
Velocity	BHWV 13A	GHWV 14A
Sitting Height	SHCB 21	SHCG 22
Sitting Height and Sub-		
ischial Leg Length	LSHB 51	LSHG 49
Biacromial Diameters	BCB 34	BCG 35
Biiliac Diameters	BIB 36	BIG 37
Triceps and Subscapu-		
lar Skinfolds	SKB 45	SKG 46
Head Circumference		
0–16 years	HCB 18	HCG 19
Gairdner/Pearson Growth		
Charts for Infants	GPB	GPG
Skeletal Maturity Score	SMB 47	SMG 48

2. Measuring Instruments

The instruments listed below are available from:
Holtain Ltd, Crosswell,
Crymmych, Pembrokeshire

Harpenden Anthropometer
Gives a direct and accurate reading to the nearest mm, over a range 50 mm to 570 mm.

Harpenden Stadiometer
Counter balanced movement giving accurate and direct readings to the nearest mm over a range of 600 mm to 2100 mm.

Harpenden Portable Stadiometer
Counter balanced movement giving accurate and direct readings to the nearest mm over a range of 850 mm to 2060 mm.

Harpenden Infant Measuring Table
Gives direct readings to the nearest mm over a range of 230 mm to 1200 mm.

Harpenden Supine Measuring Table
Gives direct readings to the nearest mm over a range 300 mm to 2100 mm.

Harpenden Neonatometer
2 standard lengths:
(a) Long: for normal neonates, measuring range 188 mm to 750 mm.
(b) Short: for pre-term babies, measuring range 180 mm to 600 mm, for use in incubators.

Harpenden Infantometer
Follow-up instrument to the Neonatometer. Measuring range 300 mm to 940 mm. Automatically locks at correct measuring point.

Harpenden Skinfold Caliper
Reads to 0.2 mm at standard jaw pressure of 10 g per mm^2. Measuring range 0–500 mm.

Holtain/Tanner–Whitehouse Skinfold Caliper
Reads to 0.2 mm at standard jaw pressure of 10 g per mm^2. Measuring range 0–480 mm.

Prader Orchidometer
Obtainable from: Professor A. Prader, Kinderspital, Steinwiesstrasse 75, 8032 Zurich, Switzerland.

Wright Peak Flow Meter
The following models are obtainable from:
Clement Clarke International Ltd,
Airmed House, Edinburgh Way,
Harlow, Essex CM20 2ED.
Standard Model. Records in 5 litres per min. divisions over a range 60–1000 litres per min.
Low Range Model. Records in 5 litres per min. divisions over a range 20–200 litres per min.
Mini Wright Peak Flow Meter. This is a recently introduced cheaper variation of the model.

3. Developmental Screening Tests

Information about these tests, including the Denver Developmental Screening Test, is available from The Test Agency, Cournswood House, North Dean, High Wycombe, Buckinghamshire.

References

Bakwin, Ruth M., Weider A. and Bakwin H. (1948) Mental Testing in Children, *Journal of Paediatrics*, **33**, 384.

Bryant, Gillian M., Davies, Kathleen J. and Newcombe R. G. (1974) The Denver Developmental Screening Test. Achievement of test items in the first year of life by Denver and Cardiff infants. *Developmental Medicine and Child Neurology*, **16**, 475.

Buckler J. M. H. (1977) Comparison of systems of estimating skeletal age, *Archives of Disease in Childhood*, **52**, 667.

Coleman J. M., Iscoe, Ira and Brodsky M. (1959) The 'Draw-a-Man' Test as a predictor of school readiness and as an index of emotional and physical maturity. *Paediatrics*, **24**, 275.

De Roo T and Schröder H. J. (1976) *Pocket Atlas of Skeletal Age*. Martinus Nijhoff, The Hague, Netherlands.

Dubowitz, Lilly M. S., Dubowitz V. and Goldberg, Cissie (1970) Clinical assessment of gestational age in the newborn infant. *Journal of Paediatrics*, **77**, 1.

Farr V., Mitchell R. G., Neligan G. A. and Parkin J. M. (1966) The definition of some external characteristics used in the assessment of gestational age in the newborn infant. *Developmental Medicine and Child Neurology*, **8**, 507.

Frankenburg W. K. and Dodds J. B. (1967) The Denver Developmental Screening Test. *Journal of Paediatrics*, **71**, 181.

Gairdner D. and Pearson, Julie (1971) A growth chart for premature and other infants. *Archives of Disease in Childhood*, **46**, 783.

Godfrey S., Kamburoff P. L. and Nairn J. R. (1970) Spirometry, lung volumes and airway resistance in normal children aged 5–18 years. *British Journal of Diseases of the Chest*, **64**, 15.

Goodenough F. L. (1926) *Measurement of Intelligence by Drawings*. World Book Co, New York.

Harvey D. and Parkinson, Christine E. (1977) When do the first teeth come through? *Journal of Maternal and Child Health*, **2**, 446.

Hodson C. J., Drewe J. A., Karn M. N. and King A. (1962) Renal size in normal children. *Archives of Disease in Childhood*, **37**, 616.

Jackson D. and Fairpo C. G. (1976) Unpublished data.

Jordan S. C. and Scott, Olive (1973) *Heart Disease in Paediatrics*, pp. 32 and 35, Butterworth & Co Ltd, London.

Marshall W. A. (1971) Evaluation of growth rate in height over periods of less than one year. *Archives of Disease in Childhood*, **46**, 414.

Marshall W. A. and Tanner J. M. (1969) Variations in pattern of pubertal changes in girls. *Archives of Disease in Childhood*, **44**, 291.

Marshall W. A. and Tanner J. M. (1970) Variations in pattern of pubertal changes in boys. *Archives of Disease in Childhood*, **45**, 13.

Parkin J. M., Hey E. N. and Clowes J. S. (1976) Rapid assessment of gestational age at birth. *Archives of Disease in Childhood*, **51**, 259.

Pyle S. I., Waterhouse, Alice M. and Greulich W. W. (1971) *A Radiographic Standard of Reference for the Growing Hand and Wrist*. Press of Case Western Reserve University, Chicago (distributed by Yearbook Medical Publishers, Chicago).

Rao D. H. and Sastry J. G. (1976) Day-to-day variation in body weights of children. *Annals of Human Biology*, **3**, 75.

Sheridan, Mary D. (1968) *The Developmental Progress of Infants and Young Children*, 2nd edn. DHSS Reports on Public Health and Medical Subjects, No. 102. HMSO, London.

Silver A. A. (1950) Diagnostic value of three drawing tests for children. *Journal of Paediatrics*, **37**, 129.

Smithells R. W. (1971) The prevention and prediction of congenital malformations. In *Scientific Basis of Obstetrics and Gynaecology*, p. 252. Ed. R. R. Macdonald. Originally published by J. & A. Churchill, London, subsequently by Churchill/Livingstone, Edinburgh.

Tanner J. M. (1962) *Growth at Adolescence*, 2nd edn. Blackwell Scientific Publications, Oxford.

Tanner J. M., Goldstein H. and Whitehouse R. H. (1970) Standards for children's height at ages 2–9 years allowing for height of parents. *Archives of Disease in Childhood*, **45**, 755.

Tanner J. M., Hiernaux J. and Jarman, Shirley (1969) Growth and physique studies. In *Human Biology: a guide to field methods*, p. 1. Ed. J. S. Weiner & J. A. Lourie. Published for International Biological Programme by Blackwell Scientific Publications, Oxford.

Tanner J. M. and Whitehouse R. H. (1973) Height and weight charts from birth to 5 years allowing for length of gestation for use in infant welfare clinics. *Archives of Disease in Childhood*, **48**, 786.

Tanner J. M. and Whitehouse R. H. (1975) Revised standards for triceps and subscapular skinfolds in British children. *Archives of Disease in Childhood*, **50**, 142.

Tanner J. M. and Whitehouse R. H. (1976) Clinical longitudinal standards for height, weight, height velocity, weight velocity, and the stages of puberty. *Archives of Disease in Childhood*, **51**, 170.

REFERENCES

Tanner J. M. and Whitehouse R. H. *Atlas of Children's Growth.* To be published by Academic Press, London in 1979.

Tanner J. M., Whitehouse R. H. and Healy M. J. R. (1962) *A New System for Estimating Skeletal Maturity from Hand and Wrist Radiographs, with Standards Derived from a Study of 2600 Healthy British Children.* Centre International de l'Enfance, Paris.

Tanner J. M., Whitehouse R. H., Marshall W. A., Healy M. J. R. and Goldstein H. (1975) *Assessment of Skeletal Maturity and Prediction of Adult Height (TW2 Method).* Academic Press, London.

Tanner J. M., Whitehouse R. H., Marshall W. A. and Carter B. S. (1975) Prediction of adult height from height, bone age, and occurrence of menarche, at ages 4–16 will allowance for mid-parent height. *Archives of Disease in Childhood,* **50**, 14.

Tanner J. M., Whitehouse R. H. and Takaishi M. (1966) Standards from birth to maturity for height, weight, height velocity, and weight velocity: British children, 1965. *Archives of Disease in Childhood,* **41**, 454 and 613.

Woods D. L. and Malan A. F. (1977) Assessment of gestational age in twins. *Archives of Disease in Childhood,* **52**, 735.

Zachmann M., Prader A., Kind H. P., Hafliger H. and Budliger H. (1974) Testicular volume during adolescence. *Helvetica Paediatrica Acta,* **29**, 61.

Ziegler R. F. (1951) *Electrocardiographic Studies in Normal Infants and Children.* Charles C. Thomas, Springfield, Illinois, USA.

Index

Numbers in bold type indicate pages on which illustrations appear